Accident and Emergency Handbook

Accident and Emergency Handbook

David H. Wilson MB ChB, FRCS, DTM & H

Consultant, Accident and Emergency Department, General Infirmary, Leeds
Senior Clinical Lecturer in Surgery, Leeds University

Michael W. Flowers MB ChB, FRCS

Consultant, Accident and Emergency Department, General Infirmary, Leeds
Senior Clinical Lecturer in Surgery, Leeds University

Butterworths
London Boston Singapore Sydney Toronto Wellington

First published 1985
Reprinted 1988

© Butterworth & Co (Publishers) Ltd, 1985

British Library Cataloguing in Publication Data

Wilson, David H.
  Accident and emergency handbook.—5th ed.
  1. Wounds—Treatment   2. Medical
  emergencies
  I. Title   II. Flowers, Michael W.
  III. Wilson, David H. Casualty Officer's handbook
  617′.1026   RD93

  ISBN 0-407-00328-2

Library of Congress Cataloging in Publication Data

Wilson, David H.
  Accident and emergency handbook.

  Rev. ed. of: Casualty officer's handbook. 4th ed. 1979
  Includes index.
  1. Wounds and injuries—Treatment—Handbooks, manuals,
etc. 2. Medical emergencies—Handbooks, manuals, etc.
I. Flowers, Michael W.   II. Wilson, Michael W. Casualty
officer's handbook.   III. Title. [DNLM: 1. Emergency
Service, Hospital—handbooks. 2. Wounds and injuries—
handbooks. WX 39 W747a]
RD93.E44 1985   617′.1   85–4169
ISBN 0-407-00328-2 (pbk.)

Photoset by Butterworths Litho Preparation Department
Printed and bound in England by Butler & Tanner, Frome, Somerset

Preface

It is almost a quarter of a century since Maurice Ellis prepared the first edition of *Casualty Officers' Handbook*. In this time Accident and Emergency Medicine has become an established specialty in Britain, North America and Australasia. Its early growth owed much to Ellis's pioneer work and its present development is a tribute to his efforts.

In the fourth edition Malcolm Hall was my co-author and his contribution was greatly appreciated. Since his retirement he has graciously passed the position of co-author on to Michael Flowers who is my fellow Consultant in the Accident and Emergency Department of the Leeds General Infirmary.

This new edition reflects the experience which Michael Flowers and I have shared over the past decade in teaching and training junior doctors in Accident and Emergency. We feel the time is right to change the title of the book in keeping with the designation and growth of our specialty and we have undertaken a comprehensive revision of the text. An additional chapter has been added on Practical Procedures. Our aim has been to provide a concise and comprehensive handbook which will guide and teach a junior doctor in the wide variety of his daily work in an Accident and Emergency Department. It is our hope that medical students and nurses will also find the book helpful.

We have sought expert help in the preparation of two of the chapters. Our thanks are due to Dr Ian Smith for revising the chapter on Paediatric Emergencies and to Dr Ivor Quest for providing an up-to-date account of legal problems in the chapter on The Accident Officer and the Law.

We also wish to express our thanks to Patricia Braithwaite for typing the text and to Peter Hargreaves and the staff of the Medical Photographic Department of the General Infirmary at Leeds for the photographic illustrations.

D.H.W.

Contents

Chapter 1

Introduction to the Accident and Emergency Department

More new patients are seen in the Accident Units of our country than all hospital out-patients put together. The number of patients has doubled in the last 25 years and equals approximately 20 per cent of the total UK population per year. Less than 20 per cent have been sent by their doctors, so the large majority present without warning and often without any previous diagnosis or assessment. Seventy per cent are classified as accidents (trauma) as distinct from acute medical and surgical conditions, which equally divide the remainder. Almost a quarter of the patients are aged between 15 and 24 years, a disproportion entirely due to the male members of the community.

Orientation

It is clear then, that as a doctor new to the A & E Unit, you will have to adjust to considerable differences in clientele and style of work from your previous post, where you were able to have a more leisured and considered approach. You will see the patient in his own clothes, at an early stage in the evolution of his condition, and you must be brief but exact in your assessment and decisive in your management. You will face sudden transition from irritation at a trivial complaint, to an overwhelming injury demanding all your resourcefulness and courage. You are likely when on duty to be busy all the time, and under pressure by the nursing staff to keep the queue moving. Therefore you need to be co-operative and pliable, firm and compassionate, well-informed and teachable.

Team-work

In no other hospital work is it so important to secure and maintain excellent working relationships with the whole range of staff, including not only nurses but porters, technicians and paramedical support services.

It is particularly important, for example, to obtain information from the ambulance personnel as to the condition and situation of the patient when first called, and to enlist the co-operation of the physiotherapist and medical social worker in the assessment of the fitness of the patient to go home.

In particular, however, dependability in turning up on time for shifts, flexibility in staying on if extra help is needed at the end of the shift, co-operation over holidays and time off, and a willingness to share out the less attractive aspects of the shop floor work are all essential.

A good relationship with the general practitioner must be fostered. His opinion will be respected, and a reply to his letter is only courteous. Where a patient is sent home after an injury or incident where supervision is necessary for any reason, you must either telephone or write to the family doctor with details of investigations and expected outcome.

The relationship with the hospital specialities is a delicate one. You will already have done recent house jobs, so that you will be familiar with the recurring problems, but the shortage of beds or the lateness of the hour or the nature of the case, for example, may combine to make certain patients' management a focus of argument. The A & E doctor must be prepared to take a strong initiative in the best interests of the patient, and, if necessary, call your senior for support; on the other hand you must also be courteous and inform the relevant resident doctors of all urgent cases clearly requiring admission, even if the patient does not require to be seen by them first in the department.

There needs to be a regular medical team meeting within the department, where cases can be discussed, where medical audit can take place and a programme of teaching pursued.

Decision making

It is important wherever possible to be decisive in both diagnosis and management, and it is particularly important to explain clearly to the patient what is happening. The provisional diagnosis and suggested management should be recorded in the notes before investigations are initiated. This is not only good practice, but if the shift ends before the investigations are complete, the doctor taking over the case gets a clear lead rather than having to start again. It is particularly important to hand over responsibility for such cases to the next team member personally whenever feasible.

You will need to cultivate a method of working that will allow the right mix of rapid but careful assessment and good judgment where unwarranted delay will be caused by superfluous investigations. You must be humble enough to accept any wisdom from the nursing staff on this point.

Note keeping

Clarity and appropriate detail must not be obscured by unnecessarily long examinations and notes. The salient features from a rapid systematic examination usually suffice. Illustrate wherever possible. Measure wounds, describe them and enumerate the stitches required. If appropriate, use photography. Obviously confidential information or remarks that could be misinterpreted should be avoided in the notes which might be read by patient or relatives. Symbols and abbreviations should only be used if clearly understood by other staff and the writing should be legible and the signature of the doctor decipherable.

Play it safe

A & E doctors are highly vulnerable, so it is important to be aware of where dangers lie. Negligence in law means a lack of expected care and attention, and A & E doctors occupy a particularly exposed position within the Health Service. Many investigations, such as a skull radiograph, may be done for defensive purposes and some patients will be admitted unnecessarily, but there is no excuse for us in law if we do not play it safe and give the patient the benefit of any doubt that exists (*see* Chapter 24). There is always plenty of back-up and you must never be too proud to call in help.

Keeping informed

There should ideally be a departmental library with 24 hour access to reference books but in any case you will need to be well instructed, even if only from a theoretical point of view, in all the possible practical procedures you will be expected to perform as they arise. In particular, intubation, cardiac massage and defibrillation will be familiar to most, if not all, A & E doctors – but even then the particular procedure followed by the department should be immediately and thoroughly learnt so that the team functions without a hitch in the event of cardiac arrest. Obviously the techniques of suturing, venous cut-down, central venous pressure access, subclavian vein puncture, arterial blood sampling, thoracic drainage, peritoneal lavage and the cricothyroid stab should be thoroughly rehearsed and understood before venturing into the resuscitation room (*see* Chapter 25). The doctor must familiarize himself early on with all the particular equipment and instrumentation used in the department, as wide variations exist between different hospitals and units.

Most doctors new to A & E work are initially apprehensive about dealing with the musculoskeletal trauma, and even, for example, minor fracture manipulation creates more fear than dealing with cardiac arrest. An alarming and important article by Yates and Wakeford* points out how few doctors before appointments in A & E departments have experience in what are essential and regularly required procedures for the Casualty Officer. It becomes vital, therefore, for there to be regular teaching and careful supervision, and persistent encouragement on the part of more experienced staff, and a follow-up clinic staffed by senior clinicians where mistakes can be picked up.

The major incident

Each department will have its own arrangements and the task of the new A & E doctor is to memorize his role in the event of a major incident, and also to examine the equipment reserved for calls to the site of incidents.

---

* Yates, D. W. and Wakeford, R. (1983). The training of junior doctors for A & E work. *Injury,* **14,** 456–460

Chapter 2

The management of the severely injured patient

At the scene of the accident

The first person to reach the victim of a serious accident may have the best chance of saving life, provided he or she is trained in First Aid.

If the injured person cannot breathe within 3–4 minutes irreversible brain damage will have occurred and all other efforts at resuscitation and treatment will fail. Care of the airway is of paramount importance.

Because serious injuries are so frequently associated with road traffic accidents, all car drivers should be trained in First Aid.

When confronted with an accident situation the steps to follow are:

1. Remove or protect the victim from further hazard.
2. Clear the mouth and pharynx of secretions, blood, vomit, false teeth or other foreign material.
3. If the patient can then breath adequately, place him in the recovery position (*Figure 2.1*).
4. If the patient cannot breath adequately, start mouth to mouth resuscitation. (A Brook Airway makes this easier and more effective; *Figure 2.2*).
5. Apply pressure to external bleeding points. Raising an arm or leg above the level of the heart will diminish venous blood loss.
6. Send someone else to alert the rescue service.
7. If there are several victims of the accident, give priority to the more seriously injured, provided they appear to have a chance of surviving.

The emergency ambulance team

1. The ambulance will be directed by radio and, in an urban situation, will usually arrive within 5 minutes.

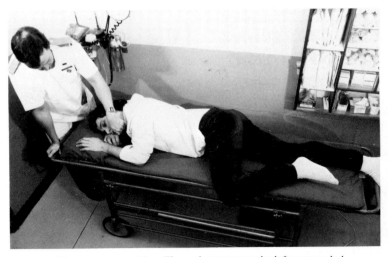

Figure 2.1 The recovery position. The patient must not be left unattended

2. The ambulance man will check the respiration. He has suction and a pharyngeal airway available.
3. If necessary, pulmonary ventilation can be supplemented by giving oxygen through an Ambu bag.
4. Entonox (50% nitrous oxide and 50% oxygen) is carried by the ambulance. It can be used to ease pain but, as with oxygen, it must not be used in the presence of fire or sparks from cutting equipment.
5. Sterile pressure dressings will be applied to control external blood loss and other wounds should be protected by sterile dressings.
6. A spinal board will be used to diminish the risk of injury to the spinal cord while extricating and moving the patient.
7. Temporary splints and bandages are supplied to support limb fractures and the patient is placed on a stretcher.
8. Details of the nature of the accident and, in a road traffic accident, the impact speed should be taken from witnesses or surmised from the state of the damaged vehicle.
9. An estimate should be made of the quantity of blood lost at the scene of the accident.
10. The Accident and Emergency Department must now be alerted by radio of the number of victims, their approximate ages, their injuries and the estimated time of arrival at hospital.

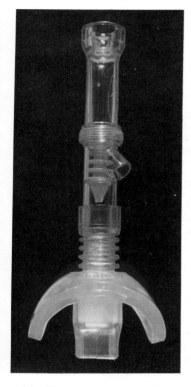

Figure 2.2 Brook airway for 'mouth to mouth' resuscitation

11. Transport of patients to hospital by either road or air should be as quick as practical without causing any further injury or distress. The patient's condition must be observed throughout the whole of the journey, special attention being paid to the airway and respiration.

General practitioner immediate care

1. A passing doctor or a General Practitioner called through an 'Immediate Care Scheme' will check the above procedures and co-operate with the rescue personnel.
2. If necessary, and if equipped, he will pass an endotracheal tube.
3. If necessary he will start an intravenous infusion.
4. He will make an estimate of the injuries and alert the A & E department.
5. The general practitioner will diagnose death in fatally injured victims.

Accident and emergency flying squad

1. The A & E Flying Squad will check the First Aid treatment and co-operate with the rescue personnel.
2. They will intubate the patient and start an intravenous infusion if necessary.
3. They will give analgesia or anaesthesia to facilitate freeing a trapped patient.
4. Under extremely exceptional circumstances they may perform an emergency amputation of a limb.
5. They will decide on priorities of evacuation and alert the A & E Department.
6. They will diagnose death in fatally injured victims.

In the resuscitation room

The resuscitation room in the Accident and Emergency Department should be warm, well-lit, private and have adequate floor space to resuscitate at least three patients simultaneously. The equipment must be readily available and in good working order (*Figure 2.3*). There should be voice communication with the whole of the A & E department and telephone communication with the rest of the hospital. The medical and nursing staff must be familiar with the type and location of each item of equipment.

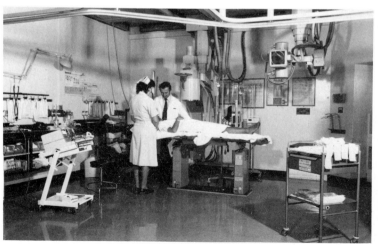

Figure 2.3 Resuscitation room with facilities for intubation, ventilation, fluid replacement, monitoring and radiology

Efficient resuscitation requires team-work. The delegation of duties among the members of the team should be done by the senior doctor. The essential procedures are listed below in order of priority, but ideally they should run concurrently.

Airway and breathing

Check the air passages, remove false teeth or other foreign bodies, suck out secretions, blood or vomit from the mouth and pharynx. Hold the jaw forward and introduce a pharyngeal airway. Apply oxygen through a face mask. If there is then any doubt about the adequacy of the patient's respiration determine the cause and, if practicable, pass a cuffed endotracheal tube. Inhaled blood or vomit, a flail chest, tension pneumothorax, ruptured diaphragm, ruptured bronchus, lacerated lung or high cervical spinal cord injury are to be considered.

If the lung and visceral pleura are lacerated, positive pressure ventilation, as when 'bagging' the patient, can rapidly produce a fatal pneumothorax. Chest drains must be introduced to prevent such a catastrophe or to decompress a haemopneumothorax. Repeated arterial blood gas analyses should be used to monitor and record the effectiveness of the treatment. For further details of the management of chest injuries, *see* Chapter 7.

Fluid replacement

To make an initial assessment of the need for fluid replacement it may be necessary to cut the clothing along the seams to avoid the trauma of undressing the patient. As this is done, baseline information is recorded of pulse, blood pressure, respiration, temperature and level of consciousness; this will be a guide as to whether fluid replacment is indicated. The ambulance attendant's report is also helpful at this point. Were the circumstances of the accident such that internal bleeding is likely? How much blood was lost at the scene of the accident and during the ambulance journey? How much blood has been soaked up by the patient's clothing and the First Aid dressings? The volume of internal bleeding into the limbs is related to the swelling. A fracture of the shaft of the femur will result in approximately one litre of blood being extruded into the soft tissues of the thigh. A major disruption of the pelvis with palpable instability may cause 2–3 litres of blood to be lost to the circulation. Similarly, the thoracic and abdominal cavities can each accommodate three or more litres of blood. The presence of such massive internal haemorrhage should always be considered when the patient fails to respond to an apparently adequate volume of fluid replacement.

If the extent of the injuries is such that circulatory collapse is likely to develop then fluid replacement must be started immediately. It is much easier to introduce a large intravenous cannula when the peripheral veins are well filled; once they have collapsed, even with a satisfactorily placed cannula, it may be difficult to obtain an adequate rate of transfusion and cannulation of the subclavian vein may become necessary.

There is no one sign, nor any single clinical measurement, on which to make a diagnosis of shock. It is a composite picture of a cold, anxious, pale, sweating patient with rapid shallow respiration, the pulse rate is raised and the pulse volume reduced, the blood pressure is low and the peripheral veins are collapsed. This situation demands immediate transfusion of warmed blood under pressure, possibly at multiple sites. A central venous pressure monitor will be useful in determining the rate and volume of transfusion.

For patients in either category, those in whom shock is anticipated and those in whom it is already present, a sample of blood should be taken for grouping and cross-matching as soon as the intravenous cannula is introduced. The quantity of blood to be requested will depend on the clinical assessment.

The first choice for the transfusion site is a forearm vein, but injuries or other circumstances may make it necessary to use the external jugular vein or a scalp vein in a baby. When the peripheral veins are all collapsed, subclavian cannulation or a 'cut-down' in the femoral triangle are indicated.

Choice of fluid

There is considerable difference of opinion as to the type of fluid to use. The choice lies between electrolyte solutions, plasma substitutes, plasma and whole blood.

Electrolyte solutions   normal saline or Hartman's solution are usually employed to establish the infusion and in less severe cases may be all that is necessary. They can also be used for fluid replacement until fully grouped and cross-matched blood is available provided pressure remains at a satisfactory level.

Plasma substitutes   can perform two functions: those containing molecules of a relatively small size (about 30 000 molecular weight) are valuable for the restoration of the peripheral circulation in tissue of doubtful viability; those with larger molecules (60 000–70 000 molecular weight) are used to maintain or restore the circulating blood volume. The dextrans have been used for these purposes for many years but they have the disadvantage of causing difficulties in blood cross-matching if given before taking the blood sample from the patient. Solutions using a modified gelatin molecule (e.g. Haemaccel) are now widely used but occasionally they cause an allergic reaction.

Plasma   reconstituted plasma may carry the risk of transmitting serum hepatitis and plasma protein fraction is to be preferred. It is expensive to produce and its use should be restricted to cases where there is a biological indication, as in the treatment of burns.

Whole blood   is preferable to other replacement fluids when the combined external and internal blood loss in a formerly healthy patient is estimated to be greater than 20 per cent of the circulating blood volume (*Figure 2.4*). Group O Rhesus negative blood is in short supply and should only be used when time does not permit cross-matching procedures to be carried out. In a severe emergency group O Rhesus positive blood can be used for male patients (or post-menopausal women) for whom this factor is less significant. The normal antibody screen on a patient's blood takes at least 30 minutes, but homologous blood, checked for ABO and Rh factor only, can be available in 10 minutes.

Full compatibility tests can take as long as 2 hours and a decision may have to be taken to use blood which has been grouped but not cross-matched. When blood is being transfused a doctor must check each unit before it is administered.

In the A & E department it is not unknown for two patients bearing the same name to be injured in the same accident, and for both to require blood transfusion. Identification must therefore include both the patient's name and the hospital registration number. The Typenex system uses a wrist band with multiple detachable sticky labels with a unique number and these can be used to identify all the patient's specimens. The response of the patient to the transfusion must be recorded at regular intervals and failure to respond will suggest continued internal bleeding.

Physical examination of the whole body

The respiration and circulation are now under control and a more detailed examination of the patient can be undertaken. The history of the accident is important. The ambulance man's account

12

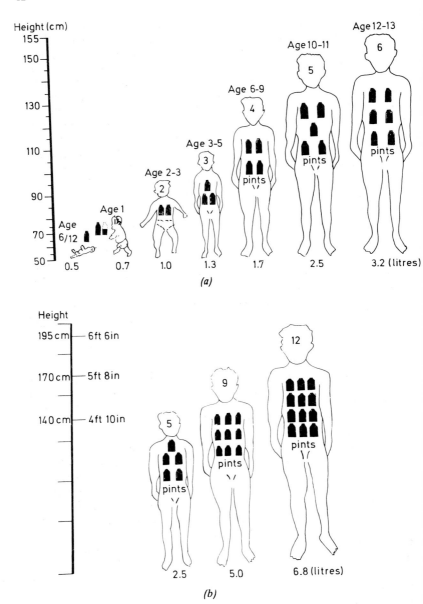

Figure 2.4(a) Average normal blood volume in children by age and height. (b) Average normal blood volume in adults by height

should allow an assessment to be made of the violence and the various forces to which the patient was exposed. Following a high velocity road accident, it is always wise to assume that the patient will have sustained a deceleration type of injury such as a rupture of the aorta, even if the initial examination is apparently normal. Imprints on the skin of a seat belt, clothing or a steering wheel must be noted and strongly suggest the likelihood of damage to internal viscera. From a clinical point of view the abbreviation 'RTA' for a road traffic accident is meaningless without further details. The type of injury sustained by a pedestrian is different from that suffered by a motor cyclist and a car driver will also have a different pattern of injury. Patients injured in explosions will probably have sustained damage to the ear drums and lungs, and this again will be suggested by the history of the accident.

Because the conscious patient does not necessarily give a comprehensive account of his symptoms he requires a full examination. The unconscious patient, being unable to guide the doctor, must be similarly examined. It is advisable in the conscious patient and essential in the unconscious patient, to repeat the physical examination at regular intervals until the extent and progress of the injuries allows the correct decisions to be made for their management. All the physical findings must be recorded and the time noted. A member of the resuscitation team can act as a scribe writing down not only the history and the details of the physical examination, but also a record of blood samples despatched and transfusions and injections given to the patient. A wall board at the head of the trolley may be used to mark up the progress of the vital signs so that the team, and any other doctors who are called in, can see at a glance how the patient is responding.

The physical examination should follow an established routine. Injuries to the head and trunk carry the greatest threat to life in the first few hours, and so are accorded priority. The presence of a spinal injury cannot be excluded at this stage and all handling of the patient must be done carefully with this possibility in mind. Details of the examination and treatment of the head, trunk and limbs are described in the appropriate chapters. The possibility of the patient having a pre-existing illness or an acute medical disorder before the accident must not be overlooked. It is also helpful to know if the patient has been drinking alcohol, was receiving medication or taking illicit drugs, as this may affect the physical signs or alter the reaction to the trauma or its treatment. After a comprehensive examination of the head, thorax, abdomen and pelvis, the nature and extent of any limb injury should be noted. When dressings and splints are applied the fingers and toes must be left exposed to allow a continuous assessment of the circulation in all four limbs. Blankets and sheets should not be allowed to hide these areas.

Ideally, X-ray examination should be done in the resuscitation room. In the unsatisfactory event of this not being possible, then the process of resuscitation and the necessary regular physical observations must continue in the X-ray Department. Recent experience with fluoroscopy and image intensification in the resuscitation room has proved to be of immense value. The integrity of the cervical spine can be demonstrated. A dynamic picture of cardio-respiratory action is obtained. Fractures, dislocations and foreign bodies are quickly located and the whole comprehensive survey takes only 1–2 minutes.

The use of drugs

A patient may have sustained a major injury but will not necessarily complain of pain. The only indication for the use of analgesia is a complaint of pain. Entonox or local anaesthetic nerve blocks will give temporary analgesia during the application of splints and well-applied splints are, of themselves, immediately effective in reducing pain. It is preferable not to use other analgesics because they may mask the patient's symptoms and possibly depress respiration. Pupillary signs will be less reliable and the level of consciousness may be modified. If further analgesia is necessary morphine in small doses (5–10 mg in an adult) can be given intravenously and the dose repeated as indicated by the patient's response. The newer synthetic analgesics have still to establish themselves in emergency care. The use of steroids in shock is slowly gaining acceptance. An intravenous infusion of methylprednisolone (30 mg/kg) given over the course of 20 minutes is claimed to reduce the incidence of the Adult Respiratory Distress Syndrome in the subsequent 2–3 days and is also used for patients in septic shock. Patients on long-term medication such as insulin, steroids, beta-blockers, digitalis, etc. will require special consideration during their resuscitation and expert assistance may be required for their management. The use of antibiotics and tetanus prophylaxis in the treatment of wounds is discussed in Chapter 18.

Arrangements for definitive treatment

Several specialist units may be involved in the management of any one patient. Priorities in treatment will be decided by these specialists, but it remains the responsibility of the accident and emergency doctor to ensure that the overall well-being of the patient is not jeopardized by excessive concentration on any one injury. The departmental routine must ensure that each patient has his own unique registration details and these should be attached to the patient by a wrist band. This registration number must be used on all forms and biological samples, and the departmental staff must make sure that the results of all laboratory investigations are transmitted to the specialists involved in the patient's definitive treatment. While the patient is receiving resuscitation in the A & E department arrangements will be made for his transfer to a ward, the intensive care unit, the operating theatre, or occasionally, to some other specialized hospital. During transfer the patient should be accompanied by a doctor or a nurse and it may be wise to have a portable suction apparatus available during the journey.

Interviews with relatives

Every A & E department should have a quiet, pleasantly furnished room where patient's relatives can wait and be told of the progress of the resuscitation and the immediate plans for the patient's treatment. The room should have a handbasin, mirror and telephone. It is important for medical and nursing staff to make sure of the identity of the people in the interview room and their relationship with the patient, before passing on personal details or catastrophic news. Similarly, information received from relatives immediately following an accident may not necessarily be accurate and, if possible, confirmation should be discretely obtained before acting upon it. The onerous task of informing relatives of the fatal outcome of an accident must be done with compassion and sympathy and is a task for the senior doctor and nurse on duty. The necessary skills for handling such difficult situations should be taught to all staff joining the department.

Chapter 3

X-rays in the Accident and Emergency Department

X-ray abuse?

Approximately 50 per cent of patients attending the department will have a radiograph. It is therefore clear that there must be X-ray facilities within the department, and if possible these must function round the clock. This is not only to facilitate the flow of such an enormous number of patients, but also to minimize the danger of transporting ill people and the extra staff and time involved in accompanying them. The trolleys used for such patients should be radiolucent as even transfer from trolley to trolley can cause deterioration in severely ill patients.

Vigilance must be maintained so as not to overuse an already pressured and expensive service. Many patients are radiographed unnecessarily. X-rays are no substitute for a careful history and clinical examination. However, medicolegal vulnerability compels care in this respect. It is better to play safe, and a clear departmental policy should be worked out to guide the doctors. The senior radiographer in the A & E section and a radiologist should be involved in teaching and should help in laying down guidelines, so that a balance can be achieved between the risk of negligence arising from withholding X-rays unwisely, and the expense and exposure to radiation involved in over-enthusiastic investigation.

The doctor needs to co-operate with the radiographer, and be open to correction if necessary. For example, she could well ask the doctor if a young woman in the second half of her menstrual cycle could be managed without radiographic examination. The patient, however, may apply pressure and this needs to be properly evaluated. The general practitioner also may send a patient just for an X-ray, and it is usually courteous to accede to such a request and send a report back with the patient.

How to request an X-ray

A good, clear, readable history and examination is helpful, particularly pointing out exactly where any tenderness is, or any entry wound of a possible foreign body, for example. Although the radiographer takes standard views of each part, he or she may, in addition, be asked to help in deciding the best angle for the particular problem in mind. The doctor should state exactly what he is wanting to visualize, and leave it to the skill of the radiographer. The latter may well have useful observations to make on the resulting film and the doctor must not be too proud to ask for advice.

How to examine an X-ray

1. An efficient viewing screen is essential. A window or a strip light in the department will not do. An auxillary high intensity light source is also advisable to reveal, for example, areas of soft tissue calcification or glass foreign bodies.
2. The doctor should satisfy himself that the film does, in fact, belong to the patient in question and that the correct side has been X-rayed.
3. A systemic examination of the X-ray begins with putting the film on the screen in its anatomical orientation. Any obvious abnormality should not prevent the doctor from carefully checking each represented system in turn, and a routine must be developed to ensure that nothing is missed (*see* below). A thorough knowledge of the normal is essential.
4. It is unwise to blame the radiographers for what may appear to be an inadequate film without first consulting with them. The patient may be obese or restless.
5. Any previous X-rays need to be found for comparison, if available, and if a limb is being examined, a radiograph of the opposite side would be advisable for comparison if any doubt exists.

What to look for

The skull and facial X-ray

1. Linear fractures need to be distinguished from sutures and vascular markings.
2. Shift can be seen if the pineal gland is calcified.

3. Air-fluid levels may be seen in the sphenoid sinus and in the frontal and maxillary sinuses, and may be the only sign of fracture.
4. Soft tissue shadowing is usually evident in the maxillary sinus following a 'blow-out' fracture of the orbital floor.

The chest X-ray

1. Is there a fractured rib(s)?
2. Is there a pneumothorax? (Views in expiration and inspiration should be requested.)
3. Is there a haemothorax? (These are best seen if the patient is vertical, but if this is impossible, then a lateral decubitus film will show them.)
4. Is there a lung contusion?
5. Is there mediastinal shift or widening?
6. Is there enlargement of the heart?
7. Is the diaphragm normal? intact?
8. Is there surgical emphysema?

The abdominal X-ray

1. Is the diaphragm normal? Is there any subdiaphragmatic air?
2. Is there blurring of the psoas shadows?
3. Are the outlines of the liver and kidneys visible? Any soft tissue shadows displacing organs, any fluid levels? (Again a lateral decubitus view is helpful if the patient cannot be erect.)
4. Is there any bowel distension?

Cervical spine X-ray

1. Can you see the whole of the cervical spine?
2. Is there any muscle spasm, straightening the normal lordosis?
3. Are the anterior and posterior aspects of the vertebral bodies in line?
4. Is the odontoid process in correct relationship with the atlas body?
5. Are the spaces between the spinous processes equal?
6. Is there any prevertebral soft tissue swelling?

Limb X-ray

1. Ensure two views, at right angles usually. Ensure the joints above and below the part are included.

2. Is the bone quality normal? X-ray of the opposite limb may be useful to avoid confusion about epiphyses.
3. Are there any displacements of soft tissues such as fat pads around joints?
4. Is a stress film necessary?

Audit

Some form of audit is wise. All X-rays should be reviewed by either a radiologist or a senior member of the A & E staff. If missed lesions are picked up the doctor responsible needs to be informed and a senior member of the staff must decide whether the patient requires to be recalled.

The mistakes arise usually from inexperience, from failure to grasp the significance of clinical evidence, or from a different doctor examining the X-rays. Staff new to the department, and particularly those working on a sessional basis, are particularly vulnerable. If in doubt clinically, the patient should be reviewed in the follow-up clinic to provide a second and more senior opinion.

Chapter 4

Head injuries

Major head injuries

The management of head injuries in the A & E department must follow a strict routine. The eventual outcome may be uncertain but the A & E procedures are clear cut and precise and are as follows.

Airway and breathing

If necessary, suck out the mouth and pharynx, lift the jaw forward and administer oxygen through a face mask. If the patient is unconscious and respiration is inadequate, pass an endotracheal tube. If facial trauma makes this impossible, perform a tracheotomy (*see* Chapter 25). If there is also an injury to the chest beware of creating a tension pneumothorax when inflating the lungs; chest drains will be required to correct this complication. Inadequate oxygenation will aggravate the head injury by increasing cerebral oedema.

Take a history

Details of the accident may be obtained from witnesses, the ambulance men or the patient. Following a road accident ask the following questions:

1. What was the impact speed? High speed injuries cause diffuse brain damage due to shearing of the brain tissue.
2. Has the patient been unconscious? The length of the period of amnesia is a measure of the severity of the head injury.
3. How long is it now since the accident occurred?
4. Have observers noticed a change in the patient's level of consciousness? Either an improvement or a deterioration is important.
5. Has the patient vomited or had a fit?
6. What is known about the patient's general health? Has he been taking alcohol, drugs or any other medication?

Physical examination

1. Examine the scalp, face and neck for bruising, tenderness, swelling, wounds, foreign bodies, bony crepitus, extruded brain.
2. Look in the ears for c.s.f. and blood indicating a fracture of the base of the skull.
3. Examine the eyes for local trauma, pupillary size and reaction to light.
4. Palpate the cervical spine for tenderness, bruising, swelling or any irregularity in the line of the spinous processes. Any positive findings may indicate that the cervical spinal cord is at risk and the patient must be moved with extreme caution.
5. Examine the mouth and throat for oral trauma and look for c.s.f. and blood leaking into the pharynx from a fractured base of skull.
6. Examine the rest of the body to detect other injuries and particularly examine for muscle tone, voluntary movements and reflexes in all four limbs.

Record baseline information

The management of the patient will be determined almost entirely by the serial recording of clinical observations. These should be done in a systematized way which is agreed by all the medical and nursing staff who will be caring for the patient. The Glasgow Coma Scale is now widely used (*Figure 4.1*). It is essential that the nurse or doctor making the recordings understands the significance of each observation and reports any deteriorating sign immediately.

Investigations

Blood gases

If there is any doubt about the adequacy of the respiration take 2 ml of arterial blood in a heparinized syringe from the radial or femoral artery. A modern, automated blood gas analyser will give a printed analysis within 2 minutes. Systems which produce results after 30 minutes or more are useless in this context; by the time the results are available the situation will have changed, but in which direction? The advantage of using an automated analyser is that a second sample can be measured 15–20 minutes after the first and the response to treatment can be evaluated.

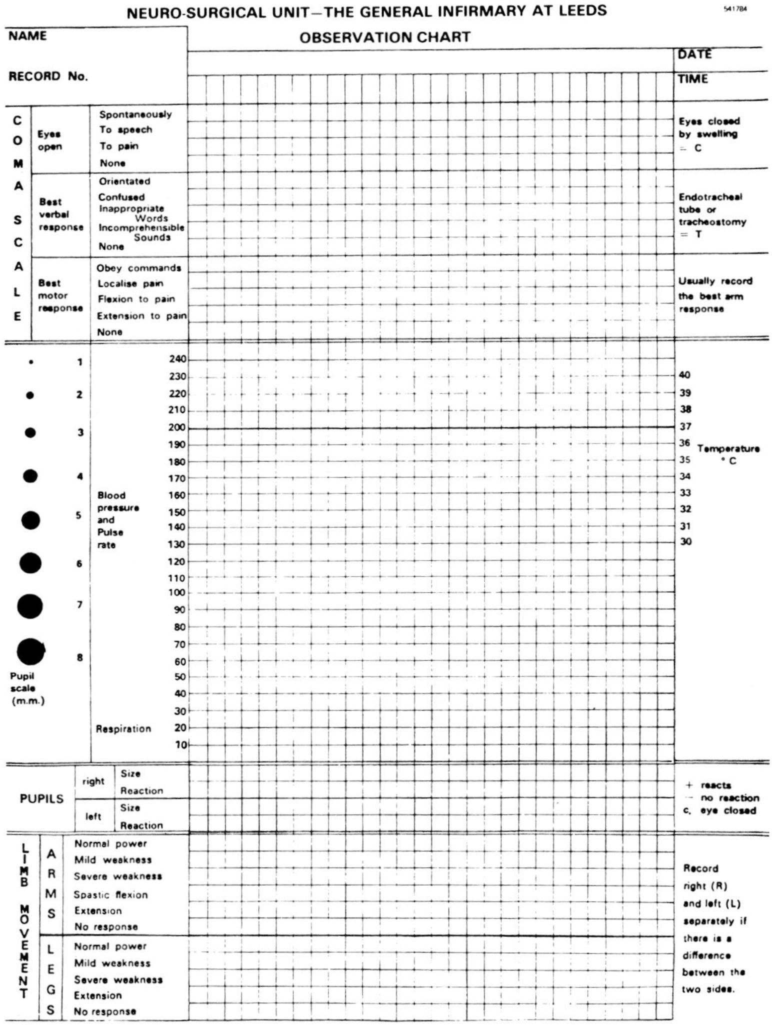

NEURO-SURGICAL UNIT—THE GENERAL INFIRMARY AT LEEDS   541784

OBSERVATION CHART

NAME

RECORD No.

DATE

TIME

C O M A	Eyes open	Spontaneously		Eyes closed by swelling = C
		To speech		
		To pain		
		None		
S C	Best verbal response	Orientated		Endotracheal tube or tracheostomy = T
		Confused		
		Inappropriate Words		
		Incomprehensible Sounds		
		None		
A L E	Best motor response	Obey commands		Usually record the best arm response
		Localise pain		
		Flexion to pain		
		Extension to pain		
		None		

Pupil scale (m.m.)
1
2
3
4
5
6
7
8

Blood pressure and Pulse rate

240 230 220 210 200 190 180 170 160 150 140 130 120 110 100 90 80 70 60 50 40 30

Respiration 20 10

Temperature °C
40 39 38 37 36 35 34 33 32 31 30

PUPILS	right	Size		+ reacts
		Reaction		− no reaction
	left	Size		c. eye closed
		Reaction		

L I M B M O V E M E N T	A R M S	Normal power		Record right (R) and left (L) separately if there is a difference between the two sides.
		Mild weakness		
		Severe weakness		
		Spastic flexion		
		Extension		
		No response		
	L E G S	Normal power		
		Mild weakness		
		Severe weakness		
		Extension		
		No response		

Figure 4.1 Glasgow coma scale

Hypoxia and hypercarbia are both accompanied by an increase in cerebral oedema and must be corrected. Arterial oxygen tension should be above 10.7 kPa and P_{a, CO_2} between 3.5 and 4.5 kPa.

Blood alcohol

The patient may smell of alcohol but it is impossible to say whether the alcohol alone has caused a significant deterioration in the level of consciousness unless it is measured. Levels below 100 mg/dl are unlikely to produce changes on the 'coma scale' but recordings over 200 mg/dl can cause coma in the absence of a head injury. If the patient has suffered an injury it must not be disregarded.

Imaging

Plain X-rays If there is an indication to X-ray the skull (*see* below) three views at least are required: posteroanterior, lateral and Towne's projections. The lateral view should also include the cervical spine to demonstrate any bony injury which might be a risk to the spinal cord. If there is any suspicion of a depressed fracture then tangential views should also be taken. A nurse must stay with a head injury patient during the X-ray examination to continue the neurological observations and to be on hand if the patient vomits or has a fit.

Linear fractures of a varying degree of complexity are the commonest abnormal finding. When a fracture line runs across the meningeal grooves in the temporal region a meningeal vessel may have been damaged and close attention must be taken for the first sign of an extradural haemorrhage.

Separation of the suture lines indicates that considerable force has been applied to the skull. It occurs more often in younger patients; in the older age group very severe violence is necessary to produce this lesion.

Patients who suffer a fracture through the cribriform area of the skull may develop cerebrospinal rhinorrhea and a traumatic aerocoele which will show on X-ray. Antibiotic therapy should be started to prevent meningitis and the patient referred to a neurosurgeon. It may eventually be necessary to close the hole in the dura and remove the fistulous track between the nasopharynx and the cranial cavity.

At the initial examination of the PA plain film a search should always be made for the pineal body: it is calcified in about 30 per cent of adults. If precise measurements with a ruler indicate that the pineal body is not central then there is probably an intracranial haemorrhage developing and neurosurgical advice should be sought immediately.

Ultrasound mid-liner If the conscious state is disturbed and the pineal body cannot be seen on the plain films, ultrasound may be used to determine whether there has been a shift of the cerebral hemispheres within the cranium. A skilled technician is required to produce reliable results, a positive finding is significant but it can be dangerous to place too much confidence in a negative result.

CAT scan   The detailed information provided by this investigation is invaluable provided the time spent on it does not over-delay the performance of a life-saving craniotomy, or compromise the maintenance of life support in a critically ill patient. The frequency with which it is used will depend on its proximity and availability.

Emergency treatment

Maintenance of the airway and adequate oxygenation remain the first priority.

If the patient is having fits, after noticing any localizing signs, the fits should be controlled. Intravenous diazepam will usually achieve this and so diminish the demand for oxygen and the tendency towards a metabolic acidosis.

Cerebral oedema, which accompanies fits, vomiting and unresponsive pupils may be diminished by an intravenous infusion of 20% mannitol, 3 ml/kg body weight being given over the course of half an hour. This will serve 'to buy time' while preparations are made to do burr holes for the evacuation of an intracranial haematoma.

Hypotension must be corrected by blood transfusion. Scalp wounds may bleed profusely. Bleeding points should be ligatured or undersewn and open wounds protected by a sterile dressing until definitive treatment can be applied. If blood transfusion does not rapidly restore the arterial blood pressure then there is probably continuing internal blood loss elsewhere in the body for which appropriate measures must be taken.

If the patient's condition has not been stabilized by the above treatment then burr holes should be made as quickly as possible to decompress an extradural or acute subdural haematoma.

If the condition is stabilized but still critical then many neurosurgeons would introduce intracranial pressure monitoring to indicate if and when further intervention is necessary.

If brain death occurs then the possibility of organ donation should be considered. The nationally agreed procedures will be initiated by the transplant team.

Minor head injuries

The distinction between a major and a minor head injury is an arbitrary one and there is always at least a theoretical risk of the minor situation developing life-threatening complications. The vast majority of patients who attend an A & E department following an injury to the head require no specific treatment and they eventually make a full recovery.

Taking an accurate history of the accident and the subsequent clinical course, followed by a general physical examination, are the essential basic steps to follow in order to decide how to manage each situation.

Children

Children constitute a large proportion of these patients. Their parents are naturally anxious. Even after a minor head injury children often turn pale and vomit. Every A & E department should have a short-stay ward where such patients can be under the close supervision of an experienced nurse for 2–3 hours until it is clear that they have recovered. Even then it is advisable to give the parents a 'Head Injury Instruction Leaflet' (*Figure 4.2*) before they take the children home.

LEEDS GENERAL INFIRMARY ACCIDENT & EMERGENCY DEPT.

INSTRUCTIONS RE HEAD INJURIES

If the patient complains of :-

DROWSINESS

ANY VISUAL DISTURBANCE

VOMITING

HEADACHE

you should contact your own Doctor or return to the Hospital

AT ONCE

Figure 4.2 Head injury instruction card

Occasionally the parents will return with the child 2 or 3 days later because it has developed a painless cystic swelling under the scalp. X-ray examination will probably reveal a linear fracture through which cerebrospinal fluid leaked to create a subgaleal hygroma. This condition is not dangerous and the patients can be reassured that the swelling will disappear in 1–2 weeks. No treatment is required.

X-ray examination

The decision to X-ray the skull after a minor head injury must be taken on the evidence of the history and physical examination. If the loss of consciousness was only transitory (less than a minute) and the patient is now fully recovered without any tenderness on palpation of the scalp, radiological investigation can be safely omitted. Anxiety is always felt because some patients have a 'lucid interval' after a head injury before they become unconscious again from the build-up of an extradural haematoma. Such patients have usually been unconscious for more than a minute following the accident and they are likely to have a headache and tenderness of the scalp on physical examination. In these circumstances radiological examination of the skull may, or may not reveal a fracture. Irrespective of the X-ray findings they should be kept under observation for a few hours.

Chronic subdural haematoma

This condition is seen either in young children or elderly patients. The young patient will have been listless and fretful and may have weakness of one or more limbs. Dilatation and conjugate deviation of the pupils may be present. Plain X-ray may show separation of the suture lines and a CAT scan will confirm the diagnosis.

The elderly patient will have suffered a marked impairment of mental faculties in the preceding 3–4 weeks. Loss of memory and confusion are accompanied by a disturbance of gait and balance. Examination may show ocular paralysis and papilloedema. The X-ray of the skull may show a shift of the pineal body and a CAT scan will demonstrate the location and extent of the lesion.

Lacerations of the scalp

The hair should be clipped and shaved for a distance of 1 cm around the wound. Local anaesthetic is injected into the wound and any devitalized tags of tissue are resected. Bleeding should be stopped by catgut ligatures and general oozing is dealt with by firm pressure. A search is made for foreign bodies such as glass from a car window and a probe should be used to detect any irregularity in the surface of the skull which would indicate that the patient has an open fracture. The galea is then sutured with catgut and the skin closed with either monofilament synthetic sutures or, for a small wound, catgut sutures which will be absorbed in 10–14 days.

If bleeding has been well controlled a dressing is unnecessary. If it is felt that oozing may occur a firm dressing can be applied for 24 hours, after which the wound should be left open. Plastic sprays, adhesive strapping or adhesive dressings should not be used. They make suture removal difficult, they will be painful to remove and they serve no useful therapeutic function.

Tetanus prophylaxis should be given when appropriate (*see* Chapter 18) and the patient, or the parents, given a Head Injury Instruction Leaflet.

Non-absorbable sutures can be removed after one week. Because of its good blood supply the scalp heals rapidly. If the initial wound toilet has been adequate and the suturing properly carried out, infection or other complications will not occur.

Many patients have intermittent headaches after even a minor head injury. They should be reassured that this is not unusual, no treatment other than simple analgesia is required and the symptoms will probably disappear within 1–2 months.

Chapter 5

Injury and emergency of the face and neck

The significance of the facial injury to the Casualty Officer lies in the danger to the airways. The further management may lie in the province of one of several specialties and the appropriate faciomaxillary team needs to be involved at an early stage.

Causes of airway obstruction

1. Accumulation within the mouth of vomit, or blood or broken teeth and dentures. These must be cleaned out with the finger wrapped in a swab, and suction used thoroughly.
2. *Swelling* of the lips, tongue or pharynx may result from direct trauma or from thermal or chemical injury. Early tracheostomy may need to be instituted.
3. *The tongue* may obstruct either by swelling or laceration or by instability induced by unconsciousness or some fractures of the mandible. These patients may be more comfortable erect, if conscious, and if unconscious will need the tongue stabilized manually or with a suture through its substance or by the semi-prone position.
4. *Facial fracture,* with displacement of the maxilla may cause direct obstruction as well as inevitable bleeding. Most bleeding will stop spontaneously, and is rarely life-threatening if the airway can be protected. The bleeding can often be controlled by direct pressure.

Injury to the nose

A blow on the nose with epistaxis suggests fracture, particularly if deformity is present. Obstruction of either nasal passage should be noted. Swelling may mask deformity, but there will be marked tenderness and the fracture is sometimes compound to the outside with a puncture wound at the bridge. Septal swelling should be looked for and noted. Bleeding stops rapidly.

X-ray examination is not essential. The problem is chiefly cosmetic, and can be assessed by external appearance. The ENT department will wish to see the patient when the swelling has diminished but before the nasal fracture has united, i.e. between 5 and 10 days after the injury.

Epistaxis, a common reason for presentation at the A & E department, is usually due to bleeding from Little's area. It is easily halted by pressure with the thumb for several minutes. Cautery with silver nitrate can be undertaken if the bleeding point is visualized, or if the patient attends repeatedly. Advice should be sought from the ENT department. If the bleeding is from further back, it may be unremitting and the cause may be hypertension. Vital signs and the haemoglobin level should be checked, and an attempt should be made to halt the bleeding by packing the nose. The conventional packing carefully done may well be sufficient but a postnasal pack or balloon catheter against which packing can be buttressed is sometimes required (*see* Chapter 25). This patient may well require admission if bleeding has been prolonged and copious, but if not the patient needs to be seen in the ENT Clinic the following day for removal of the pack.

Injuries to the teeth

Avulsed teeth can be replaced. The patient should be encouraged to find and bring missing teeth, but care must be taken not to miss an inhaled tooth and if there is any doubt, follow-up X-rays must be arranged. An expiratory chest film gives maximum information.

Bleeding tooth sockets are a common source of referral to the A & E department, and the Casualty Officer should pack with adrenaline-soaked gauze. If this fails, the pack can be retained by suturing the gum over the gauze and the patient referred back to the dentist (*see* Chapter 25).

Injuries to the tongue and mouth

Small lacerations can be left without repair, but larger lacerations will bleed repeatedly and cause distress to the parent and patient alike. Suture can usually be performed with local anaesthesia using absorbable suture material. Lacerations of the palate may require a general anaesthetic if extensive, or in a child or in an unco-operative patient.

Lacerations of the face

Obviously, the utmost care must be taken to produce a cosmetically acceptable result. Layers must be accurately repaired. Alignment of the tissues must be meticulous so that there is no resulting step, for example, in either lip margin or eyebrow.

Local anaesthetic may distort the tissues and confuse the picture, so that regional nerve blocks such as the supra-orbital, infra-orbital and inferior dental blocks allow more exact assessment and repair.

Much of the suturing in the department may be done by medical students or nurses but complex facial lacerations should be referred to either a plastic surgeon or a senior member of staff.

Dogs bites are not uncommon around the mouth and have potential for producing unpleasant infection which may well compromise the cosmetic result. Antibiotic cover must be given, and careful and judicious wound excision carried out. The same is true for deep abrasions where tattooing is feared. Scalpel excision or brushing must be carried out with appropriate anaesthesia.

Through and through lacerations of the lips caused by penetration of the teeth also may become infected, and these wounds should be repaired both inside and outside. If a tooth is totally or partially missing, X-ray examination must be undertaken to decide if a fragment is retained within the lip. The same is true of glass injuries to the face, although since the introduction of seat belt legislation such injuries are uncommon.

Injury to the ear

Lacerations which involve cartilage require careful reconstitution, suturing the skin but not the cartilage.

Haematoma (the Rugby player's ear) requires assiduous aspiration urgently, followed by pressure pads shaped to the contours of the ear, shaped out of orthopaedic felt and bandaged or strapped pressing the ear against the head. This needs to be repeated every day or so until there is no re-accumulation of haematoma. If control is not achieved, the ENT department should be consulted about the possibility of more elaborate surgical drainage.

Rupture of the eardrum may occur with a blow to the side of the head and once the diagnosis is confirmed no further measures are required except to warn the patient not to allow water into the meatus. The ear should not be packed and no ear drops are necessary; the patient is referred to the next ENT Clinic.

Injury to the facial skeleton

The middle third

This comprises the central maxilla, nose, ethmoid and the related sinuses. Fractures can be grouped into three predictable types, classified by Le Fort, as illustrated in *Figure 5.1*.

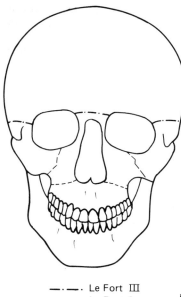

—·—· Le Fort III
----- Le Fort I
— — — Le Fort II

Figure 5.1 Le Fort classification of injuries to the middle third of the facial skeleton

Le Fort I

This is caused by a blow to the maxilla, severing the tooth-bearing portion of the maxilla from the rest of the facial skeleton. This segment is mobile but produces minimal deformity and will manifest itself clinically by epistaxis, damage to the dental surface and teeth, and crepitus on manipulation. It does not directly endanger the airway.

Le Fort II

This is clinically obvious if displaced as the 'stove-in' face. The middle third of the facial skeleton becomes detached and is usually driven backwards and downwards, thus compromising the airway and producing an open bite.

Le Fort III

The fracture extends into the anterior fossa through the cribriform plate and c.s.f. rhinorrhoea may be seen. The face is elongated.

These patterns may combine in differing permutations, and making an accurate assessment requires faciomaxillary expertise. There is nearly always gross facial swelling and periorbital ecchymosis. Bleeding within the mouth and pharynx may be considerable. The Casualty Officer must clear the airway and keep it clear by suction, positioning and if necessary endotracheal intubation. With severely comminuted injuries it may be appropriate to manipulate fragments into a more favourable position as a temporary expedient.

The Malar complex

This comprises the lateral maxilla (*Figure 5.2*) and zygomatic arch. The injury is a direct blow to the cheek and displacement inward is common. No immediate danger threatens and the advice of the faciomaxillary team can be sought at leisure.

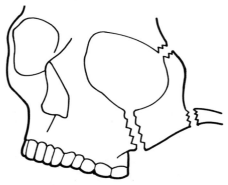

Figure 5.2 The Malar complex

Undisplaced fractures are diagnosed by subconjunctival haemorrhage extending posteriorly into the fornix, and opacity of the affected maxillary antrum. The patient should be asked about anaesthesia of the upper teeth and lip of the affected side. These patients should be referred to the faciomaxillary surgeon.

The 'blow-out' fracture

This important injury results from a blow in the orbit with the pressure created pushing orbital contents through the floor of the orbit into the maxillary antrum. The only evidence may in fact be a 'tear-drop' of soft tissue appearing on X-ray hanging down into the antrum, but in more severe injury, enophthalmos is detectable and diplopia on looking upwards may be observed due to tethering of the peri-orbital tissues. The importance lies in the permanent diplopia that may result if fibrosis of the inferior extra-ocular muscles is allowed to take place. The orbital contents are replaced and the orbital floor repaired, when indicated.

The mandible

A blow on the chin may cause direct bony injury at the site, or indirect fracture near the temperomandibular joint. Careful examination of the subcutaneous border should reveal localized tenderness. The fracture, if in the tooth-bearing area, is likely to be compound into the mouth. Mobility, and a disturbed occlusion is simple to test. Extensive comminution may destabilize the tongue and airway problems are then present.

X-ray examination is best carried out with an Orthopantomograph (*Figure 5.3*) and early referral to a Dental Service is therefore required.

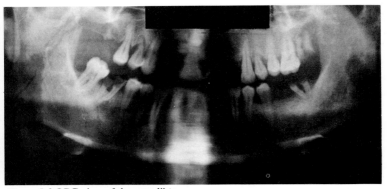

Figure 5.3 OPG view of the mandible

Dislocations of the jaw

These are easy to diagnose as the mouth is always propped open painfully. It is often recurrent. The treatment is simple but requires usually some form of analgesia and sedation. Diazepam is useful in this respect and only rarely is there need for recourse to a general anaesthetic. The two thumbs, guarded with swabs or gloves, are placed in the patient's mouth over the back teeth and steady downward pressure is applied, at the same time levering the point of the chin upwards with the fingers of both hands. Providing the patient is conscious and it is not a recurrence, no further measures are required.

The *temporomandibular joint dysfunction syndrome* is a fairly common cause of attendance, usually in young women. The painful clicking they experience may be aggravated in the presence of malocclusion and other dental problems and the dental surgeons will be happy to see such a patient. X-rays of the temporomandibular joint need practice to interpret and are not usually necessary in this condition.

Injury to the soft tissues of the neck

These may be closed, such as in a blow from an assailant, or a seat belt injury, or they may be open such as in a self-inflicted throat laceration or when pitched through a windscreen and lacerating the pharynx or larynx.

These are rare injuries but, particularly in closed truama, any skin markings of the neck must be noted and vigilance maintained to keep the airway unobstructed.

Immediate endotracheal intubation may be necessary but may be rendered impossible by tissue distortion and displacement or profuse bleeding, and tracheotomy or cricothyroidotomy may be required urgently. This is best done in the emergency situation by pushing one or two 12-gauge Medicut or similar needle and cannula through the cricothyroid membrane in the mid-line (*see* Chapter 25). This obtains some respite while a more considered approach is decided upon, presumably a formal tracheostomy by experienced staff. The traditional stab with some form of knife is hazardous, particularly in small children, and should not be attempted. If the pharynx is lacerated, surgical emphysema is evident and may embarrass the airway further. Urgent repair is required.

The foreign body

The range of things that children and adults contrive to swallow or inhale or insert into the nose or ear is astonishing. Dental equipment or broken pieces of teeth or glass, or pins and safety pins as well as the traditional pea and sweet, may all be inhaled. Coins and bottle tops, razor blades and bed springs and many more bizarre objects are swallowed accidentally or deliberately and may get stuck.

The oropharynx

The commonest foreign bodies presenting as having lodged are fish or meat bones or coins. The former will stick in the back of the tongue, the pillar of the tonsils, the tonsils themselves if present, or in the vallecula. The coin, however, may lodge at the entrance to the oesophagus and produce alarming distress. Often the foreign body has, in fact, passed but symptoms continue to arise from abraded mucosa.

X-ray investigation will be useful when the material is radio-opaque but fish bones are often disappointing in this respect. If there is an obvious oesophageal obstruction but the foreign body is not visualized, an emergency barium swallow is unwise as oesophagoscopy then becomes impossible.

To examine the back of the tongue and pharynx the tongue tip is grasped in a swab and held while light via a head mirror allows a hand free to manipulate forceps. Indirect laryngoscopy with a mirror is a skill the Casualty Officer does well to acquire and will allow the whole of the pharynx to be visualized. However, if the foreign body is present the distress so caused will probably encourage the doctor to enlist the help of a more experienced colleague.

The nose

These are usually problems of childhood, and present with precise detail from the parent; occasionally the complaint will only be of a unilateral foul-smelling discharge.

If the child is amenable, the parent helpful, and the foreign body visible via the speculum, removal may be attempted by the Casualty Officer with either a hook or suitable forceps after spraying the mucosa with cocaine. If success is in doubt it is better not to try, but to refer to a more experienced colleague, as the child may well permit only one attempt.

The ear

The object is likely to be easily visible, but great care should be taken not to push it further in. Its exact nature and shape should be researched if possible and unless it is near the external orifice and can easily be hooked out, it is probably best to refer for expert attention. General anaesthesia is sometimes needed, particularly because most of these patients are small children.

An intriguing recent fashion is the impacted and often infected *earring*. Rarely is there a need for anaesthesia. While the stud is grasped in artery forceps to steady it, the 'butterfly' at the back of the ear is gently coaxed off the pin using fine artery forceps which may have to be introduced into the substance of the pinna to find its buried wings. The earring is then withdrawn painlessly.

Chapter 6

Eye emergencies

The care of eye emergencies is an important part of any Accident
and Emergency Department. In some cases the treatment needed
is beyond the skills of the unit, but the Accident Officer must be
aware of those conditions which present as acute emergencies and
which may require urgent specialized management if the patient's
vision is not to be jeopardized.

History

An accurate history is essential. In many cases the diagnosis can be
made on the information supplied by the patient and examination
serves as confirmation. The mode of onset of the presenting
symptoms is important; a sudden pain coming on, for example,
when grinding metal, suggests a foreign body. Itching suggests an
allergic condition – has there been any recent change in the make
of cosmetics used by the patient? Sudden loss of vision suggests
arterial disturbances. Gradual loss of vision, associated with pain,
suggests glaucoma.

Examination

Visual acuity should be assessed. This is essential, even if only
crude methods are used. When simple methods, such as reading a
book or a newspaper, suggest impairment, then test type should be
used. All layers of the eye should be inspected and the shape and
reactions of the pupils noted. Ophthalmoscopy is carried out when
there are indications, such as disturbances in visual acuity, that
there may be disturbances in the function of the posterior ocular
structures.
  The eyes should be examined from the front. Adult patients can
sit; children, who are usually co-operative if a parent is allowed to
hold their hand, are easiest to examine if they lie on an

examination couch, but sedation or a general anaesthetic may be necessary in an urgent situation. The examiner should stand or sit on the same side of the patient as the injured eye.

A suitable lamp, giving a well focussed, cool beam is essential and a binocular magnifier with a headband is also essential. Practice is necessary to acquire familiarity with the apparatus.

The cornea should always be stained when the history or examination suggests that the epithelial covering may be damaged. A drop of fluorescein is placed in the eye or the impregnated end of the paper strip is placed in the lower conjunctival sac for a few seconds. The fluorescein stains corneal defects a bright green, which can be seen very clearly in a blue light or in a narrow beam of well focussed light directed obliquely across the cornea.

Eye injuries

Lacerations

The treatment of lacerations around the eye follows normal practice. In all but the smaller wound, local anaesthetic should be used. Fine atraumatic suture material should be used and accurate skin apposition, without distortion of the tissue, obtained. The vascularity of the tissue makes excision of small skin tags unnecessary. When there is tissue loss, the patient should be referred to a plastic surgeon.

The eyebrows should never be shaved; this makes it difficult to resuture the skin with the necessary accuracy and may cause a permanent distortion of the eyebrow. When the wound is above the eyebrow and involves the underlying muscles, these should be sutured with catgut to avoid subsequent drooping of the eyebrow.

Wounds which involve the edges of the eyelids should be referred to the Ophthalmic Department for repair. This is especially important in those which involve the medial margins of the lids where there may be damage to the lacrimal canaliculi.

Contusions

The degree of swelling resulting from blunt trauma is frequently large enough to make inspection of the eye a difficult task, but whenever possible it should be inspected for evidence of corneal damage or haemorrhage into the anterior chamber. If possible, the vision should be assessed. A subconjunctival haemorrhage suggests a malar fracture.

It is usually impossible to feel the lower margin of the orbit, and X-ray examination will be necessary to exclude a fracture of the zygoma or a 'blow-out' fracture of the floor of the orbit. This important complication may give rise to diplopia due to trapping of the inferior rectus and inferior oblique eye muscles in the fracture; this was discussed further in Chapter 5.

If it is impossible to assess diplopia at the time of the injury, the patient, in the absence of X-ray evidence, should be re-examined after 5 or 6 days by which time the swelling will have subsided. The presence of a fracture or diplopia is an indication for the referral of the patient to the Maxillo-Facial Department. The uncomplicated case should be treated by the application of chloramphenicol eye ointment.

Subconjunctival haemorrhage is commonly seen as a spontaneous feature without trauma, usually in the elderly. Although alarming it is harmless and requires no treatment.

Foreign bodies

Intraocular

Intraocular foreign bodies should be suspected if the history suggests that the object had a high velocity when it hit the eye. The use of a hammer and chisel, turning metal on a lathe or drilling metal with high-speed drills are still situations which can cause penetrating injury and, even if there is no external evidence of injury, X-ray and opthalmoscopic examination are essential. Even if all the findings are negative, if the doctor still feels that there is a reasonable probability of an intraocular foreign body being present, he should refer the patient to the Ophthalmic Department.

Subtarsal

The patient who presents at the door of the department with a handkerchief pressed to the eye and with a history that something blew in the eye a few minutes previously will probably be suffering from a subtarsal foreign body. The eye looks irritable, blinking is painful but no foreign body can be seen.

The upper lid must be everted to show the foreign body. It is carried out by asking the patient to look downwards while the eyelashes are gently held and pulled downwards initially and then forwards and upwards around the upper margin of the tarsal plate, which is depressed either by a finger, a matchstick or a glass rod. The foreign body is removed by wiping with a moistened (saline) pledget or cotton wool wrapped around a wooden spill and the patient experiences instant relief.

Corneal

While these are generally painful, it is by no means infrequent for patients to report to the department with only minor discomfort from a foreign body which has clearly been present for 2 or 3 days.

Local anaesthetic is essential to remove any foreign body embedded in the cornea. Two or three drops of 1% amethocaine should be given into the lower conjunctival sac. A binocular loupe fixed to a headband is essential, and a lamp designed for the purpose should be used. Ordinary bulbs in reflectors are very hot and uncomfortable to the patient. If the foreign body has only been *in situ* for a short while, it may be possible to remove it with a cotton wool bud (cotton wool twisted around the end of an orange stick) moistened with local anaesthetic or saline; if it does not detach easily, removal should be continued with the point of a 38 × 0.8 mm hypodermic needle. The needle should be held at an oblique angle to the cornea to avoid impaling the tissues if the patient should move the eye suddenly. The foreign body is removed with the point of the needle and, if it becomes loose and lies on the cornea or lower conjunctiva, it should be wiped away with a moistened cotton wool bud. If it is deeply embedded and cannot be completely removed without causing further damage, the attempt should be abandoned and the patient referred to the Ophthalmic Department for further treatment.

Rust rings remaining after removal of the foreign body should be left for 3 or 4 days; after this time they are easily removed with the point of a needle.

After removal of the foreign body, chloramphenicol ointment and a short-acting mydriatic should be inserted and an eye pad applied. With a superficial foreign body the pad can be removed after 4 hours, but when a large crater has been left, healing will be quicker if the pad is kept on for a few days and eye ointment is inserted twice a day.

Corneal abrasions

These are frequently caused by children scratching their mother's eyes, by twigs when gardeners are cutting hedges or during the intial stages of wearing contact lenses when the patient attempts to wear the appliances for a longer time than the eye will tolerate. Eyes exposed to a blast of high pressure from a compressed air line may exhibit foreign bodies or multiple abrasions. Corneal abrasions and foreign bodies cause similar symptoms. Fluorescein staining is necessary to demonstrate the presence of an abrasion which will heal quickly after treatment with chloramphenicol drops or ointment.

Contact lenses should not be handled by the doctor. They are expensive, easy to lose and are best handled by the patient. If the patient does not possess a suitable container, then it is wise to ask the patient if one provided by the department is suitable. Once such a lens is lost, it is unlikely to be found again and unnecessary acrimony is easy to avoid by judicious forethought.

Flash burns

A superficial keratitis caused by exposure to ultraviolet light is common in welders (arc eye), and is occasionally seen in persons who do not wear goggles when using a 'sun-ray' lamp at home. The condition comes on a few hours after exposure and causes pain, lacrimation and photophobia. Fine superficial pinpoint staining may be seen after using fluorescein.

Pain, which may be severe, can be relieved by local anaesthetic drops. Treatment consists of applying chloramphenicol eye ointment and a mydriatic followed by an eye pad if only one eye is affected. The patient should be advised to rest in bed and report back to the hospital the following morning, by which time the majority of symptoms should have resolved. Sedatives may be necessary for the first few hours.

Hyphaema

Haemorrhage, visible in the anterior chamber of the eye, occurs after direct injury and varies from a slight brownish red deposit around the lower rim of the cornea to a marked and obvious haemorrhage occupying the whole of the anterior chamber. Once it has been diagnosed the patient should be admitted to hospital for rest and, if necessary, paracentesis of the anterior chamber.

Burns

Thermal lesions

Thermal lesions of the eye are commonly found in association with similar lesions of the face. While the patient is in the department, drying of the cornea may be prevented by covering the eye with a single sheet of thin polythene, held in place by adhesive strapping. These patients should always be referred for an ophthalmic opinion, even if the Plastic Surgery Unit is also involved. It is preferable not to apply ointment before the patient is seen by the Eye Department in order to avoid distorting the appearance of the cornea and making the area slippery and difficult to handle.

Chemical burns

These usually arise from industrial sources but the car owner may splash battery acid in his eye and the housewife may splash caustic oven cleanser in her eye.

Injuries due to caustic substances cause much greater damage than those from acids; nevertheless treatment for both groups is similar. If the eyes have not been irrigated before the patient arrives at hospital, the eyes should be immediately irrigated with tap water. If the chemical contamination is severe, the head should be immersed under water and the eyelids forced apart. Subsequently, the eyes should be profusely irrigated with large volumes of normal saline after the instillation of local anaesthetic. This process is simplified by using transfusion bottles and giving sets instead of the old-fashioned undine.

The irrigation fluid should be directed on all areas of the eye, using an eyelid retractor under the upper eyelid to allow irrigation of the superior fornix of the conjunctiva.

Fluorescein staining may reveal corneal damage and, if this is more than minimal, the patient should be referred to the Eye Department.

Lime

This injury may be caused by wet plaster or cement dust. When the eye has been irrigated before arrival at hospital and no particles of the chemical can be seen, treatment follows the methods indicated above. When the patient arrives with the substance still in the eye, after the instillation of local anaesthetic the substances should be removed with eye buds, a spud, a needle or forceps. Irrigation is then carried out and the patient referred to the Eye Department.

Penetrating wounds of the cornea

These injuries are usually easy to recognize and are frequently associated with prolapse of the iris. This causes an eccentric or ovoid pupil, associated with a small amount of black iris tissue protruding through the laceration. The anterior chamber is collapsed. A pad and bandage should be lightly applied and the patient referred to the Ophthalmic Department for admission.

Lacerations of the conjunctiva

Small lacerations heal rapidly. If there is any retraction of the conjunctiva, the patient should be referred to the Eye Department for suture.

Tetanus prophylaxis

This should not be overlooked in open wounds of the eye.

Eye infections

Eyelids

Blepharitis

This causes soreness and crusting of the lid margins. Antibiotic and steroid ointments are prescribed. Allergic inflammation can be caused by antibiotic ointment and steroids are then used alone.

Stye

A stye presents as a pointing boil on the lid margin, and is treated with local antibiotic ointment and hot bathing.

Meibomian cysts within the tarsal plate may become inflamed and cause discomfort. A discrete nodule is visualized inside the lid margin and incision and currettage is required. This is done in the Ophthalmic Department.

Dachrocystitis

This presents as a painful swelling at the inner canthus of the eye against the side of the nose, and there is usually a history of watering of the eye. The patient is commonly elderly. Antibiotic therapy is given (incision is avoided if possible), and the patient is referred to an Ophthalmic Clinic.

Conjunctiva

Conjunctivitis

Allergic conjunctivitis may produce rapid chemosis (oedema), and both steroid and antihistamine eye drops are instilled hourly until the condition settles. Referral is wise.

Bacterial or viral conjunctivitis produces a red eye which is often unilateral. There is discharge and pain, but no visual disturbance. These are contagious and hands must be carefully washed after examination. Antibiotics are best administered as drops every hour until the condition settles. If florid, a swab should be taken for culture.

Keratitis

Pain is prominent. When associated with conjuntivitis, white spots are seen on the surface of the cornea, and treatment is as for the conjunctivitis.

If ulceration is revealed by fluorescein staining, it may take a branching form. This is the *dendritic ulcer* caused by the herpes simplex virus. Steroids must not be used. Drops of 1% idoxuridine may be commenced and the patient referred promptly for specialist advice.

If the ulceration is localized, resulting from an infected abrasion, or exposure keratitis, or a recurrent infection, look for pus in the anterior chamber. If the eye cannot be seen by an Ophthalmologist immediately, a swab is taken, antibiotic and mydriatic drops are instilled, a pad is applied, and the patient referred.

Iritis

Pain and redness begin spontaneously and are associated with photophobia and sometimes visual disturbance. There may be keratic precipitates, and occasionally pus in the anterior chamber (Hypopyon) on inspection. Immediate referral is required, but if there is to be any delay, mydriatic and steroid drops are used.

Herpes zoster

There is a danger to the eye when the ophthalmic division of the 5th cranial nerve is involved. Secondary infection may follow the skin eruption and keratitis, iritis and secondary glaucoma may result. Mydriatic drops, steroid and antibiotic ointments are applied and frequent inspections in a Specialist Unit are required.

Glaucoma

This may present in an A & E department as a painful, inflamed eye. Vision is reduced. The cornea is hazy, the pupil dilated and fixed, and the eyeball feels tense on palpation.

Temporarily, pilocarpine 4% eye drops are commenced hourly, but prompt referral is indicated.

Painless loss of vision

A sudden painless profound loss of vision suggests *retinal artery occlusion*. A gradual or partial loss of vision suggests *central retinal vein occlusion,* or *vitreous haemorrhage,* or *detachment of the retina.* Hypertensive retinopathy, macular haemorrhages, and vitreous opacities (floaters) may also present in this way to the Casualty Officer. The loss of vision may be part of a neurological disorder such as a cerebrovascular accident. Urgent ophthalmic advice will naturally be sought.

Chapter 7

Injury to the chest

Injury to the chest may take the form of blunt trauma or a penetrating wound. The most common, serious multiple injuries in UK practice occur as a result of a road traffic accident and a chest injury is present in a third of all fatal road accidents. Probably one in ten of such deaths is principally due to the chest injury, and because it presents as only part of a complex problem more dramatic trauma distracts attention from an insidious but life-threatening chest condition. Thus chest injury must always be considered as a possibility and specifically looked for.

Blunt chest trauma is also a prominent feature in falls from heights, crushing injury and explosions, although these events are relatively uncommon. Penetrating injury will, in the main, be due to stabbing or a missile wound, but such an event is still uncommon in civilian UK practice.

Immediate measures

Attention to the airway

This is discussed fully in Chapter 2.

Visual inspection of the chest wall.

Clothing is removed to allow inspection of the front and back.

1. All skin markings are significant and they are carefully noted: their relationship to the mechanism of injury is determined if at all possible by reference to police, ambulance officers, or the account of witnesses. For example, if the car driver's body has deformed the steering wheel he is presumed to have a severe chest injury until proved otherwise. This visual examination extends, of course, to include markings such as the imprint of clothing on the abdominal wall and around the head and neck.

   Traumatic asphyxia produces a dramatic visual result; when there has been a severe compressive force to the

abdomen and chest, the upper trunk and head and neck are a violaceous hue and covered with petechial haemorrhages. Specific chest injury and diaphragmatic rupture must be excluded.
2. Respiratory excursion is watched both for rate and range and particularly for inequalities between right and left sides such as in the paradoxical movement seen when there is a unilateral unstable segment of chest wall with multiple fractures of ribs.

Assessment of vital signs

These will need to include, besides pulse and blood pressure, a careful note of the JVP and the heart sounds. The possibility of cardiac tamponade from contusion or rupture must be borne in mind, and an ECG is an added diagnostic aid. There is, however, no specific ECG change for cardiac contusion and a normal ECG does not exclude damage to the myocardium. If the shock syndrome is present a venous line, preferably via a subclavian venepuncture, is established, and the patient's cardiac function is continuously monitored. Blood is taken for grouping and cross-matching, but not from the arm in which any intravenous line is running, and intravenous plasma expanders are given until the blood is available. The quantity ordered and the rate of infusion will be governed by the diagnosis and the progress of the patient. As soon as practical an indwelling balloon catheter is placed within the bladder, and the urine output measured and monitored.

Continuing respiratory distress

If there is *continuing respiratory distress* despite a clear airway the following measures should be undertaken:

1. Any open wound is closed immediately with a sterile pad.
2. The chest wall is palpated for fracture or instability and also for surgical emphysema. A flail segment can be supported temporarily by hand or by a suture through the skin or round a rib, or a towel clip at the centre of the segment held manually until definitive measures are taken. Endotracheal intubation and positive pressure ventilation will be used early in such a case but this may not be possible immediately in a conscious patient in whom a full neurological assessment is necessary. Pain relief with nerve blocks will be used at a later stage.

3. *Pneumothorax* is looked for: The suprasternal notch is palpated to detect tracheal shift, resonance is percussed and the typical change in breath sounds is detected by auscultation. If tension is suspected drainage must be instituted without delay and radiographic confirmation is not obligatory; a medium bore intravenous needle and cannula is simply introduced through the second intercostal space in the mid-clavicular line and the hiss of escaping air confirms the diagnosis. Formal intercostal drainage with underwater seal (*see* Chapter 25) can then be established.

4. X-ray examination. If the condition of the patient permits it an erect AP film is taken. This must be attempted if at all possible, but if not a horizontal beam film is taken with the patient recumbent on his unaffected side and this will display fluid levels.

5. Arterial blood is obtained for gas analysis (*see* Chapter 25).

6. A swift systematic examination is carried out before endotracheal intubation is performed with particular attention being paid to the patient's neurological status, and, of course, much valuable symptomatic information may be obtained from a conscious patient.

Absence of vital signs

The patient who arrives in the resuscitation room *without vital signs,* but who was noted to have vital signs immediately prior to arrival, requires an *immediate thoracotomy* if staff are on hand who are prepared to tackle it, particularly when a known injury such as a penetrating wound is present. At thoracotomy it will be possible to clamp the root of a bleeding lung or to diagnose a ruptured aorta or, if no blood is present, to open the pericardial sac to relieve tamponade. If none of these three conditions is present the aorta is clamped above the diaphragm until the abdomen can be opened to locate the source of bleeding.

These measures are exceptional in UK practice but the relevant equipment must be available in or near the resuscitation area and staff must be instructed in its use.

Failure to improve

As a result of the intial endeavours, the patient should have improved, and this will allow a more leisurely search for further injury. Failure to improve, however, means that a significant diagnosis has been missed. This will be due usually to massive and continued bleeding from a hitherto undetected source and evidence of this will be found in a *low central venous pressure.* This may be due to an intrathoracic lesion, such as a ruptured aorta, or from an abdominal source such as a lacerated liver. It may also be due to massive retroperitoneal bleeding from a fractured pelvis. Appropriate chest and pelvic X-rays and peritoneal lavage will determine further action.

A *high central venous pressure* indicates cardiac tamponade, or pump failure due to, for example, a cardiac infarction that caused the accident in the first place. A chest X-ray may show an enlarged heart shadow, and pericardial aspiration (*see* Chapter 25) will confirm the presence of blood. An ECG may be helpful and suggest myocardial contusion. Mediastinal tamponade arising, for example, from aortic rupture will be revealed by serial erect chest X-rays and urgent preparations for an aortogram are then made.

If the oligaemia has been reversed, and no tamponade is found but the patient *continues to deteriorate,* an intracranial injury is presumed and relevant measures are instituted (*see* Chapter 4).

Specific injury

Minor chest injury

Chest wall pain

Chest wall pain of a muscular origin is common and presents frequently with a history of minor indirect trauma in a manual worker, or some recent overuse. It is particularly noted in the pectoral and interscapular areas and only requires reassurance and a course of an antiflammatory agent.

Contusion

Contusion of the chest wall is one of the commonest reasons for delayed attendance following injury. A minor blow to the chest is at first disregarded but either because of failure to resolve in a few days or because of a sudden increase in discomfort following some muscular effort, the patient is alarmed and seeks reassurance that no fracture is present. Pain can, in fact, be severe but is clearly related to the activity of the muscle groups arising from that area of the chest. It is not necessary to radiograph the chest, although that is often why they have come. Providing there is no pneumothorax clinically, symptoms can be minimized by both analgesics and adhesive strapping applied to the affected hemicircumference of the chest. All significant symptoms settle within three weeks.

Minor rib fractures

Minor rib fractures will include a maximum of three rib fractures without any other significant injury or complication. Patients usually attend hospital immediately but again it is probably not necessary to X-ray for confirmation of rib fracture as it is obvious clinically and such information does not alter management. However, if there is any suggestion of haemo- or pneumothorax, chest films in inspiration and expiration should be requested. If no immediate or chronic pulmonary lesion is present, adhesive strapping applied to the chest wall around a hemicircumference predictably provides pain relief. The fracture site can also be infiltrated by local anaesthetic, and conventional analgesic drugs are supplied. Breathing exercises are taught if there is fear of chest infection and a follow-up visit is arranged for a further radiograph.

If, however, the patient is elderly, debilitated, or has a pre-existing lung disease, it may be wise to admit to hospital. The presence of multiple fractures, or surgical emphysema, or undue distress moves the patient into the next category.

Major chest injury

Sterno-clavicular dislocation

Sterno-clavicular dislocation or fracture of the medial limit of the clavicle is usually a minor injury, when the clavicle overrides the sternum. Only symptomatic treatment is required. If, however, the clavicle underrides the sternum, injury to the great vessels must be looked for.

Sternal fracture

This is usually obvious clinically and a lateral X-ray will confirm it. It may well be innocent, particularly in the elderly, but it may be associated with injury to the underlying heart and great vessels.

Major rib fracture

Upper rib fractures often denote a severe injury frequently associated with shoulder girdle injury and the neurovascular status of the relevant limb must be examined.

Unstable segments. A 'flail' segment is clinically evident, the affected side falling during inspiration instead of rising with the other side. Care must be taken not to miss a bilateral lesion, making both sides behave similarly, or an anterior unstable segment where multiple fractures have occurred on both sides of the sternum. Such injuries are readily palpable, and initial measures have been outlined above.

Lung injury

Damage to lung tissue by the fractured ends of ribs can cause bleeding and leakage of air. However, severe lung damage can occur in the absence of fracture. Pulmonary contusions, the development of the adult respiratory distress syndrome (ARDS), infection and fat embolization are all well recognized problems that may manifest themselves without evidence of chest wall injury.

Haemopneumothorax.   This is diagnosed by clinical and radiological means and drainage is instituted as described in Chapter 25. The urgency of this measure is dictated by the state of the patient, and the presence of tension. A large amount of blood may accumulate in the pleural space and the amount drained must be measured. It needs to be remembered that at least 500 ml needs to be present to be radiologically obvious. Profuse continuous bleeding from the drainage tube calls for an urgent opinion from a thoracic surgeon and arrangements are made to cross-match at least 20 units of blood. Transport of the patient is facilitated by the use of a Heimlich flutter-valve in the drainage circuit allowing the underwater seal to be detached, but this, of course, does not allow monitoring of the quantity of blood expelled.

Surgical emphysema.   An alarming 'Michelin-man' syndrome can be produced by subcutaneous leakage of air which can embarrass the airway. X-rays are necessary to observe mediastinal air. No specific measures are required but careful observation for embarrassment of the airway is continued.

Pulmonary contusion.   Early evidence of this may be seen on the first supine chest X-ray with mottling of the lung field and serial films must be taken, the second within half an hour of the first. In conjunction with serial blood gas analysis and considerations arising from other injuries, endotracheal intubation and oxygenation are performed early to minimize the risk of atalectasis, and many favour high dosage steroids at this point (2 g in an adult).

Fat embolism syndrome.   It is unlikely that the fulminating form of this will overtake the patient while still in the resuscitation area but rapid and efficient immobilization of skeletal injury and enthusiastic oxygenation may attenuate its effects.

Rupture of the diaphragm

The left side is usually affected and is associated with sudden abdominal compression such as by a seat belt. The chest X-ray is diagnostic but must be erect and may show abdominal contents rising into the thorax. The mechanical effect of this space-occupying lesion is to compress the lungs and early ventilation via endotracheal intubation will usually be necessary.

Injury to the trachea or bronchus

This is a rare injury and the cause will be a seat belt injury to the neck which may divide the trachea in the neck, or a penetrating injury either to the neck such as in a suicide attempt, or across the chest as in gunshot or stabbing wounds.

The patient will present with gross surgical emphysema and a haemopneumothorax, possibly bilateral. When this is drained a continuous air leak will be observed and the patient will be cyanosed with respiratory distress. Diagnosis will rest on visualization at emergency bronchoscopy. Emergency tracheotomy for damage to the cervical trachea will be performed as described in Chapter 25.

Injury to the oesophagus

This may be part of a complex injury following penetration by missile or blade, but may also occur as a result of intraluminal impaction of a foreign body such as a bone, or during endoscopy, or due to sudden increase in violent abdominal compression or vomiting where the cardia is incompetent. Penetration of the wall of the oesophagus is accompanied by a severe tearing chest pain radiating to the back and mediastinal surgical emphysema.

The unpleasant results of mediastinitis make early diagnosis essential and endoscopy or barium swallow examination will locate the lesion.

Injury to the heart and great vessels

Any patient with evidence of a severe blunt or penetrating wound to the central portion of the chest posteriorly or anteriorly must be suspected of having injured the heart or aorta until proved otherwise. It must be remembered that it is possible for a patient subsequently shown to have ruptured the thoracic aorta to be brought in initially with very little to show for it. Any skin markings are noted, together with details of the mechanism of injury. Serial observations of the vital signs are mandatory, and repeated erect chest films ordered.

Stab or missile wounds.   If the knife is *in situ* the temptation to remove it must be resisted. Survival after stab wounds even to the heart are not unknown, but survival following gunshot or other missile injury to the heart is much more unlikely. Immediate thoracotomy may allow the defect in the myocardium or aorta wall to be plugged with the finger while the patient is transported to the operating theatre. If there is a sucking wound in the chest wall this is simply closed with the hand or an adequate dressing.

Apart from direct visualization in the unusual circumstances alluded to above, an aortic rupture can be confirmed by transfemoral aortography.

Aortic rupture.   It is estimated that over one in ten fatalities following car accidents are due to aortic injury. The vast majority of those who survive long enough to be seen in the A & E department will have a lesion just distal to the origin of the left subclavian artery, at the junction between fixed and mobile segments of the aorta. Survival as far as hospital also indicates that complete shearing has not occurred. The outer layers of the vessel prevent immediate exsanguination, but it is only a matter of time before rupture occurs, and as aortography is decisive it must be arranged immediately. Cardiopulmonary bypass is likely to be required and an early diagnosis is essential to allow preparations to be made.

Cardiac contusion.   This may present as low output failure and ECG abnormalities will be present. Care must be taken in an isolated injury to bear in mind the possibility of the clinical picture being due to a cardiac infarction which may have been the cause of the original accident. Care will be necessary to avoid over-transfusion by monitoring the CVP and tamponade must be excluded as a cause for the clinical heart failure.

Cardiac tamponade.   This will be caused by leakage of blood from the injured ventricles and if the pericardium is intact or has only a small wound the tamponade will prevent sudden death. The patient is hypotensive, has a high CVP and the heart sounds are masked. A large heart shadow is evident on X-ray and aspiration confirms the diagnosis and temporarily relieves the situation. Urgent thoracotomy is arranged. *Intra-cardiac* damage is rare, but valves or septa may be damaged and the heart sounds will be abnormal.

Summary

1. Check the airway.
2. Relieve a tension pneumothorax.
3. Plug a sucking wound.
4. Support a flapping segment.
5. Assist ventilation.
6. Establish a central line.
7. Replace blood.
8. Summon skilled assistance.

Chapter 8

Abdominal and pelvic trauma

Injuries to the abdomen neatly divide themselves into 'open' and 'closed'. Every open wound and closed contusion is significant enough to justify physical examination.

Open injuries

As a result of increasing urban violence, civil disturbances, bomb explosions and terrorist activities, open wounds of the abdomen are becoming more frequent. The wound and foreign bodies within it may well have forensic importance. They must be accurately described and all foreign bodies must be preserved. Nevertheless it is rare for a patient to arrive with a prolapsed bowel, and a recent penetrating injury or stab wound of the abdomen may look quite innocent on the surface. What matters is not the *length* of the skin wound but its *depth* and direction. A small wound of the bowel will produce very few symptoms until peritonitis develops several hours later, by which time the patient may have left hospital if the implications of the skin wound were not appreciated. These remarks apply particularly to gunshot wounds. A radiological examination in the erect position will not only show metallic foreign bodies but may also reveal free gas under the diaphragm if the bowel has been damaged. If the X-ray examination is negative, after exploration and suture of the skin wound, the patient should be kept under close scrutiny on the observation ward for 4–6 hours before being discharged.

Closed injuries

Any patient who complains of abdominal pain after a blow on the abdomen, especially if he vomits, must be examined and observed because of the risk of a ruptured viscus. The condition is most common in young men but can occur at any age. Road traffic accidents, work accidents, sport or play accidents, falls and assaults are the main causes, listed in descending order of frequency.

History

If the patient can recall and describe the injury this may give a lead as to the possible damage. A steering wheel blow into the upper abdomen may rupture the liver or spleen or crush the small bowel or pancreas against the vertebral column. The length of time since the injury occurred is also important; it may take up to 4 hours for the symptoms to become definite. After this time the only remaining risk of undeclared symptoms is from delayed rupture of the spleen which is described later.

Physical examination

This begins with *inspection*. Remember to assess the whole patient, looking particularly for evidence of trauma to the head and thorax as well as the abdomen. Pulse, blood pressure and especially respiration should be examined and recorded with a note of the time at which the observations were made. The shocked patient with suspected internal blood loss demands a blood transfusion. A good intravenous line should be established in the upper limb before attempting to decide whether the bleeding is into the thorax or abdomen or both. Marks on the skin of the chest or abdomen from the imprint of clothing are very significant–they imply severe trauma and visceral damage is extremely likely; but their absence is of no significance. The presence of bruising should be noted. Measuring abdominal girth is of little value. Increase in the circumference of the abdomen due to internal bleeding is a late and variable sign and can be misleading.

Palpation

This will elicit localized tenderness and should include 'springing' the pelvis and palpating the pubic rami. Blood loss from a fractured pelvis can be profuse and this injury is frequently associated with other abdominal trauma, especially rupture of the diaphragm when excessive force has produced a 'blow-out' of the abdomen. While palpating the abdomen, enquiry should be made about radiation of the pain and specific questions should be asked about pain felt behind the shoulders. Bruising or tearing of the diaphragm or damage to the liver or spleen frequently produce referred pain to the back of the respective shoulders.

Percussion

If testing for 'shifting dullness' indicates that there is free fluid in the abdomen following trauma, one can assume that the fluid in question is blood. With the patient lying supine, a ball-point pen is used to make a mark on the skin where the percussion note changes from resonant to dull as the percussing fingers pass from the umbilicus to the loin. The patient is then turned on his side and after a minute the examination is repeated, this time percussing from the upper loin towards the umbilicus and beyond. Again the point of change from resonant to dull is noted. A distance of more than 5 cm between the first and second marks is significant.

Auscultation

Probably the most important single physical finding following trauma to the abdomen is absence of the bowel sounds. No conclusions can be drawn if they are heard, but if, after listening carefully for 2–3 minutes, no sounds are heard the patient must at least remain under observation. Most significant of all, if the bowel sounds were intially present but subsequently disappear, visceral damage is likely.

Investigations

Urine

Macroscopic haematuria is diagnostic evidence of renal injury if there is pain and tenderness in the loin. The urine should always be tested for the presence of albumin or sugar. Recent experience in the use of an 'amylase stick' has shown it to be a valuable screening test. A negative result indicates that the serum amylase is not raised. A positive result should be checked by a formal serum amylase estimation. A level above 1.000 Somogyi units implies that the pancreas has been damaged and such an injury is often accompanied by damage to the overlying mesentery and small bowel.

Blood

Haematological examinations, other than grouping and cross-matching, are not particularly helpful in the acute stage.

Haemoglobin and haematocrit levels are essential as baseline information, but the rate and quantity of blood replacement is better monitored by the patient's clinical response and the readings from a central venous catheter.

X-ray

Radiological examination will reveal fractures of the pelvis or the lower ribs which encase the liver and spleen. There will be a loss of the psoas shadow on the supine film if there is a large haemoperitoneum or a large retroperitoneal haematoma. The erect film will show air under the diaphragm if the gut is torn or, 2–3 hours after the injury, fluid levels in the bowel if damage to the mensentery has devitalized a portion of the gut. Rupture of the diaphragm may be demonstrated by the presence of loops of small bowel in the chest.

Peritoneal lavage

This procedure will show evidence of a haemoperitoneum due to a rupture of the spleen or liver, and the aspirate can also be used to demonstrate a raised amylase level. The technique is described in Chapter 25. It should not be used if the patient is pregnant or if there has been a previous mid-line laparotomy.

Management

Patients with a haemoperitoneum from a ruptured liver and/or spleen require an urgent laparotomy. The operating surgeon must decide between the time to be spent on initial resuscitation and the need for immediate surgery.

In less severe injuries the diagnosis may not be immediately obvious and the decision on whether or not to operate may only be taken after a period of observation. Pulse, blood pressure, respiratory rate, abdominal tenderness and the presence of bowel sounds should be recorded at 15 minute intervals. During this time the patient may be managed on the A & E observation ward and after 3–4 hours one of three patterns will have emerged:

1. A slow, steady deterioration–laparotomy is indicated.
2. The observations, although not normal, have remained unaltered. Admission to a surgical ward for observation should be arranged.
3. The observations have remained or returned to normal. Preparations can be made for the patient to return home.

Abdominal injury as one of multiple injuries

From what has been written it must now be obvious that if there are other dramatic injuries, such as a dislocated hip or an open fracture of the leg, there is a risk that the patient may already be under a general anaesthetic for treatment of these peripheral injuries before the presence of an intra-abdominal lesion can be fully appreciated. Yet it is the slowly developing visceral lesion which may kill the patient rather than the bone sticking out through the trouser leg. All surgeons treating injured patients must be aware of the risk of central trauma being overlooked because of the more obvious peripheral injuries, and above all they must be cognisant of the responsibility they take when arranging for a general anaesthetic to be given to a patient who has been recently injured. An anaesthetized patient cannot complain of increasing abdominal pain and all the vital signs will be confused by the surgical act and the anaesthetic.

Delayed rupture of the spleen

One unsolved problem in the management of abdominal injury patients is what to do about delayed rupture of the spleen. If a patient sustains a blow over the spleen, there is a small subcapsular haemorrhage; the splenic area is tender but the vital signs are unaffected. After a period of observation the tenderness begins to subside and the patient goes home. Days or even weeks later the spleen may tear open and the peritoneal cavity fills with blood. Urgent transfusion and splenectomy are required to save the patient's life. This late presentation may be less dramatic with left upper quadrant pain referred to the shoulder tip. An ultrasound scan will demonstrate the presence of a perisplenic haematoma and this investigation can be repeated at intervals of a few days to determine whether the shadow is increasing or decreasing in size. A tethered left diaphragm or an enlarged splenic shadow following trauma to the upper abdomen should either result in an exploratory laparotomy or else advice should be given to the patient not to travel far from skilled surgical care in the subsequent 2 months.

Trauma to the urinary tract

Macroscopic haematuria in a patient who is tender over the kidney following trauma is to be regarded as diagnostic proof of a ruptured kidney. All such patients should be admitted to hospital;

nearly all of them can be managed conservatively. An intravenous pyelogram will demonstrate the degree and severity of the damage. Occasionally, if the haematuria is massive or persists for many days, renal surgery will become necessary.

The ureters are well protected from blunt trauma but rarely a stone lurking in the renal pelvis is dislodged during a traumatic episode and enters the ureter producing the classical picture of renal colic. The management and treatment is the same as for other patients with ureteric calculus.

Rupture of the bladder

Intraperitoneal rupture is usually a late night injury. Someone who has drunk too much alcohol has an overfull bladder and staggers in front of a motor vehicle. The distended bladder bursts emptying urine into the abdominal cavity. The patient arrives at hospital with severe lower abdominal pain and may well be shocked.

Extraperitoneal rupture is more common and is a complication of fracture of the pelvis. This injury of itself is less shocking to the patient but he may have an urgent desire to urinate. Despite repeated efforts no urine is produced, but a drop of blood may emerge at the external meatus. Gradually it becomes obvious that urine is being extravasated into surrounding tissues. Both forms of rupture can be confirmed by retrograde cystoscopy and they require urgent surgical repair.

Rupture of the urethra

This is also mentioned in Chapter 14 when discussing fractures of the pelvis, but urethral rupture may also be caused by falling astride a hard object. Pain, bruising and swelling in the perineum and a drop of blood appearing at the external meatus suggest the diagnosis which can be confirmed by radiological urethrography. Recent opinion is that suprapubic catheterization is preferable to attempting to pass a urethral catheter as the latter may compound the injury and also introduce infection.

Chapter 9

Injuries to the back and neck

Patients come to the Accident and Emergency Department with disorders of the back and neck for one of two reasons:

1. They have been involved in a violent accident.
or 2. They have had a sudden spontaneous onset of pain.

In either group there may be few physical signs and, of course, in the unconscious patient there are no symptoms. This means that the doctor who manages these patients must have a clear understanding of the nature of the conditions and a definite routine to follow.

Spinal injuries

These follow violent accidents and include one or more of the following elements:

1. A fracture of the bones of the spine.
2. Tearing of the ligaments which give stability to the spine.
3. Damage to the spinal cord.

Causes

Falls from a height: such as from a roof, a ladder, scaffolding, a tree or head forwards downstairs.

Objects falling onto a patient: such as bags of cement or corn, packing cases or drums falling onto the shoulders when the spine is flexed.

Road traffic accidents: although traffic accidents often produce multiple injuries, the patient may have been thrown out of the car or off a motorcycle and have suffered only an injury of the spine.

The whiplash injury is an acute cervical strain caused by a shunting accident in which a vehicle is struck from behind and the patient probably has no head restraint. The onset of pain may be delayed. The sudden hyperextension causes damage to the anterior musculoligamentous structures and protective muscle spasm rapidly produces the typical symptoms. The X-ray will show splinting of the neck by muscle spasm and possibly a small fragment of bone pulled from the antero-inferior margin of a vertebral body.

Sports injuries: particularly the contact sports such as rugby, but diving may also cause injury to the spine.

Routine of management of a patient with suspected spinal injury

Any patient who gives a history of an accident similar to those listed above and who complains of pain in the neck or back, and particularly if he complains of numbness or tingling in the arms or legs, should be managed in the following way:

1. If the patient has not been brought in on a trolley, he must be helped onto one and required to lie down immediately, even if he considers that one is making an unnecessary fuss.
2. Adequate 'manpower' should be available (doctors, nurses, porters, students, ambulance men) so that the patient can be eased up gently from the trolley as the clothes are being removed. The patient must not be allowed to sit up.
3. While this manpower is available a carrying sheet should be inserted under the patient if this has not already been done. The patient is turned very gently onto one side and the rolled-up carrying sheet is placed over half the trolley. While the patient is in this position, the spine and posterior ribs are palpated for points of tenderness. The patient is then rolled gently onto the other side so that the carrying sheet can be unrolled to cover the rest of the trolley. Carrying poles are now inserted so that the patient can be lifted onto the X-ray table and into bed without risking further damage to the spine.
4. If a lesion of the cervical spine is suspected, a reliable assistant should stand at the head of the trolley and exert gentle traction on the neck with one hand under the chin and the other hand under the occiput. After all movements for undressing and examination of the patient have been completed, the head is wedged between sandbags.

Further clinical examination

For spinal cord damage.   Reflexes and movements should be checked in both upper and lower limbs to detect signs of paralysis. Fractures of the long bones may prevent a complete test of movements, but movements of wrist and fingers, ankles and toes can nearly always be achieved even in the presence of fractures. If any sign of paralysis is discovered, cutaneous sensation to pin prick should be tested, and areas of anaesthesia noted.

For further injuries.   If the patient has multiple injuries, the routine as described in Chapter 2 should be carried out.

X-ray examination

In the resuscitation room, X-ray examination is greatly facilitated by the use of fluoroscopy and an image intensifier to scan the spine. If such equipment is not available, then the whole spine must be X-rayed and films developed and the radiological examination must not be abandoned when the first lesion is found. It is often difficult to obtain a lateral view of the seventh cervical and first thoracic vertebrae because they are obscured by the shoulders. The radiographer may require assistance to pull down on the arms and lower the shoulders so that these vertebrae can be clearly seen in this view.

Scrutiny of X-ray films

Cervical region.   The following observations should be made:

1. On the lateral view, examine the anterior border of the body of each vertebra for any sign of wedging or collapse or detachment of a small piece of bone. The 'tear drop' fracture from one corner of the anterior border of a vertebral body usually signifies that there has also been an avulsion of the anterior longitudinal ligament and possible rupture of the intervertebral disc.
2. Now examine the alignment of the posterior borders of the vertebrae. Normally this line makes a gentle continuous curve. A straight cervical spine indicates muscle spasm and this may be the only radiological evidence of neck injury. An abrupt change at one level in this curved line or a step from one vertebra to the next, is evidence of a subluxation. Remember that the bones do not need to be fractured for there to be a potentially disastrous, unstable lesion if the

ligaments are torn (*Figure 9.1*). Minor degrees of instability will be demonstrated by flexion and extension films taken under medical supervision when the original X-rays do not show any abnormality.

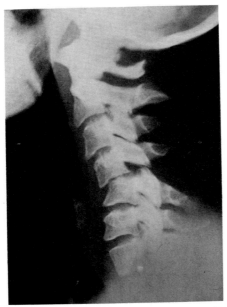

Figure 9.1 Dislocation of the cervical spine without any bony injury

3. The neural arch of each vertebra and the intervertebral joints should be examined next. If there is any doubt in the interpretation of the films, oblique views will be helpful, especially because they demonstrate any damage to the interfacetal joints. Finally, on this view, look for the rare occurrence of a fractured spinous process.

4. The antero-posterior (A-P) view should show a regular symmetrical alignment of the vertebrae. An A-P view through the mouth must always be included to show the odontoid process and the atlanto-axial joints. Special scrutiny of the base of the odontoid process should be made for signs of fracture, the relationship of the atlanto-axial joints to the odontoid process must be symmetrical, and the relationship of this process to the arch of the atlas must be checked on the lateral view.

Thoracic and lumbar regions.   The following should be looked for:

1. On the lateral view, search for a wedge-shaped collapse of a vertebral body. Old people, or those on long-term steroid therapy, may already have one or more collapsed vertebrae due to osteoporosis, so it is important to correlate the radiological appearance with the physical signs. If a suspicious wedge-shaped vertebra is found at the upper or lower border of the X-ray film, another view should be taken with the suspected vertebra in the centre of the film.
2. Examine the laminae and spinous processes for evidence of fracture. Look for a defect of the pars interarticularis especially between L_5 and S_1 (spondylolysis) or one vertebral body slipping forwards on another (spondylolisthesis).
3. The A-P view may reveal the collapse of a vertebral body. More often there is a scoliosis of the spine centred at the point of fracture. If such a scoliosis exists, the lateral view must be scrutinized again to ensure no fracture at this point has been missed.
4. In the lumbar region each transverse process of the vertebrae should be inspected in turn for fracture.
5. Finally, any ribs visible on the X-rays should be examined individually for signs of fracture.

Initial treatment of spinal injuries

Fractures of vertebral bodies and subluxation

Without paraplegia.   The management of these patients depends not so much on the bony injury itself but whether or not the spinal cord is at risk. The patient who has suffered the partial collapse of one vertebral body should be told that the injury is minimal. Such a patient will only require bed rest for 7 to 10 days followed by a similar period of physiotherapy. In consultation with the orthopaedic surgeon a decision may even be taken to manage the patient at home and so avoid admission to hospital. Conversely, the patient with a potentially unstable fracture or even a slight degree of subluxation following a ligamentous injury requires the utmost care and attention from the A & E department doctor. Responsibility for such a patient includes supervising his transport to the ward and handing him over personally to the orthopaedic surgeon or to a senior member of the nursing staff on the ward.

With paraplegia. Patients who have sustained damage to the spinal cord, irrespective of the X-ray appearance, are best admitted without delay to the Spinal Injuries Unit if this can be arranged. Only if the transfer of the patient will be delayed for several hours should the bladder be catheterized, and this procedure should be done under full aseptic conditions after telephone consultation with the staff of the Spinal Injuries Unit. During the initial period before transfer, the patient must be turned at 2 hourly intervals to avoid developing pressure sores.

Fractures of the transverse processes of lumbar vertebrae

It is important that the term 'fractured spine' should never be used for these patients. In all of them the urine should be examined for macroscopic haematuria to find out if the injury has also produced a rupture of the kidney. In the absence of this complication the patient can be told that he has bruised his back or that a very small piece of bone has been pulled from his spine. He will need bed rest and possibly analgesic tablets for a week followed by a week or two of rehabilitation, and should be able to return to heavy work within a month. It will be much longer if the patient thinks he has a fractured spine or has 'broken his back'.

Spontaneous pain in the neck and back

Patients with acute pain in the neck or back attend Accident and Emergency Departments every day. To avoid missing the few patients who have a serious condition, it is necessary to examine them all. It will speed up the process if those with cervical or thoracic pain are stripped to the waist before the doctor sees them, and those with lumbar pain are undressed as far as their underclothes and lying on a trolley.

Acute wry neck or torticollis

This well known condition often occurs as a patient is getting out of bed or dressing in the morning. It occurs at all ages and in both sexes. The head is held with the chin pointing to one shoulder. Attempts to twist the head to the opposite side causes acute pain and spasm in the neck. Physical examination should first exclude an underlying ear or throat infection. Then the muscle spasm can be relieved by using a cold 'pain relieving' spray applied over the neck muscles on the side away from the chin until the first sign of frostiness appears. As the neck warms again, the patient is instructed to move it freely. A soft collar may be worn for 2 to 3 days if the neck is still uncomfortable.

Cervical spondylosis

Degenerative changes in the cervical spine are increasingly common beyond the age of 45 to 50 years. The condition may have been symptomless until it is brought to light by a trivial blow or twisting injury, or a road traffic accident. In other patients the pain develops spontaneously. If there is pressure on the cervical nerve roots there may be pain referred to the arms, the shoulder region or between the shoulder blades. Often the patient only complains of the referred pain and is surprised by the suggestion that the root of the trouble is in the neck.

Physical examination must include noting down the range of movement in the neck in the six directions of: flexion, extension, rotation to right and left, and lateral flexion to both sides. If pain is referred to the arm, reflexes, muscle power and joint movement should be examined and compared with the opposite arm and the findings recorded. X-ray examination will very probably show the degenerative changes in the cervical spine, but the radiological appearance often bears little relation to the severity of the symptoms.

Treatment

In consultation with orthopaedic colleagues, the A & E department staff may undertake the early treatment of these patients. The principles of treatment are rest, pain relief and measures to improve the circulation and thereby probably to reduce the oedema around the nerve roots. Rest for the neck is provided by applying a cervical collar which is adjusted to hold the head in the most comfortable position. It is important for the patient to be able to sleep, and if he is more comfortable in the collar he should wear it through the night; analgesic tablets should also be prescribed to ensure sleep. By the end of the second week the patient should start to wean himself off the collar by wearing it a little less on each successive day. If symptoms persist, physiotherapy is indicated. Traction and/or manipulation of the neck help some patients but seem to exacerbate the symptoms in others. Diapulse therapy is proving to be a valuable means of easing the pain in the neck, presumably by dispersing the oedema around the nerve roots.

Low back pain

This common complaint is usually provoked by lifting with the back flexed. It may be due to a muscle strain or to ligamentous damage or, occasionally, to a prolapsed intervertebral disc.

Physical examination

While the patient is lying down, test for reduction in straight leg raising; only if the range is less than 60° is it of real significance. Examine the knee, ankle and plantar reflexes. Test for weakness in extension or flexion of the big toes, and for diminished sensation in the legs or feet. Because the pain may be partially related to the hip joint, test the range of movement in both hips. If the patient can stand, look for scoliosis, kyphosis and the loss of the normal lumbar lordosis. Palpate the spine for local tenderness and test the movements of spinal flexion, extension, lateral flexion to left and right, and rotation.

X-Ray examination

This should be done more to exclude bony abnormality, disease or secondary deposits than for any direct help in diagnosis because, as in the neck, degenerative changes often bear little relation to the severity of the symptoms.

Treatment

In low back pain the sheet anchor is rest in bed on a firm mattress. This can usually be arranged at home. Occasionally, for the patient with a prolapsed intervertebral disc, an orthopaedic surgeon may prefer to admit the patient to hospital for bed rest, traction, analgesia and further assessment with a view to laminectomy. In the rare cases of a central disc prolapse producing urinary retention, urgent operative treatment will be necessary, but by far the majority of patients will be treated by conservative methods. Following a period of bed rest, rehabilitation in the Physiotherapy Department will speed up recovery. Supervised exercises in a pool heated to 35°C is probably the most beneficial single form of treatment. Traction, manipulation, graded exercises and electrotherapy may all have a part to play. Finally, weight reduction and regular physical exercise, particularly swimming, are to be recommended to diminish the risk of recurrent attacks of low back pain.

Chapter 10

Pain in the shoulder

For a comprehensive examination of the shoulder, the patient should be undressed to the waist. The examination must include a search for evidence of nerve or vascular damage in the affected arm and also a check on the movements of the cervical spine, because of the possibility of pain being referred from the neck.

The following are the principal causes of pain around the shoulder:

Injured patients

1. Fractures of clavicle, scapula or humerus.
2. Dislocations of the shoulder, acromioclavicular or sternoclavicular joints.
3. Tears of the rotator cuff.

Uninjured patients

1. Subacromial bursitis (painful arc syndrome).
2. Supraspinatus tendinitis.
3. Pericapsulitis (frozen shoulder).
4. Referred pain.

History

Has there been a significant injury or did the symptoms arise spontaneously? What was the nature of the injury? A direct blow or a fall on the outstretched hand can cause a fracture or dislocation. A wrenching or traction type of injury can damage the soft tissues, nerves or vessels. Beware of the patient who has serious injuries elsewhere, or who is unconscious and consequently does not draw attention to his shoulder injury.

Physical examination

With the patient undressed to the waist, follow the standard sequence of Look, Feel and Move.

Look

Lacerations and bruises will be noted. If three or more days have passed since the injury occurred, a fracture of the neck of the humerus or a rotator cuff injury may have produced the characteristic pattern of bruising which only comes to the surface below the insertion of the deltoid muscle and then extends downwards towards the elbow.

A haemarthrosis arising from a fracture involving the shoulder joint produces an obvious painful swelling. Associated venous damage will cause swelling of the limb and an arterial injury will result in a blanched, cold arm.

An abnormal contour to the shoulder will suggest a fracture or dislocation. An anterior dislocation causes the shoulder to lose its normal, rounded contour as the deltoid muscle hangs vertically donwards from the edge of the acromion. The rare 'luxatio erecta' is diagnosed on site as the patient arrives with the injured arm held above the head. Prominences over the acromioclavicular or sternoclavicular joints suggest dislocation of the respective joint.

Feel

Areas of tenderness should be precisely localized and related to anatomical structures, and this may be diagnostic for a rotator cuff injury. Areas of reduced cutaneous sensation must also be recorded. Always test for damage to the circumflex humeral nerve which innervates the skin on the lateral aspect of the upper third of the arm. If it is damaged, it is important to record the finding before any manipulation is performed to prevent the area of anaesthesia and partial paralysis of the deltoid being attributed to the manipulation rather than to the initial injury. The quality of the radial pulse should be compared with that in the uninjured arm.

Move

Following a recent injury it may be impractical to ask the patient to move his shoulder but it is essential to establish that there is no motor deficit in the hand, as would be caused by a lesion of the brachial plexus.

For the 'non-trauma patient' accurate recording of the range of flexion, abduction, external rotation and internal rotation of the shoulder may be diagnostic and will form a baseline from which to measure subsequent progress. A painful arc of movement as the shoulder passes from 60°–120° of abduction establishes a diagnosis of subacromial bursitis as the bursa is squeezed between the head of the humerus and the acromion process. In the acute stage of pericapsulitis or frozen shoulder any movement of the shoulder joint will be painful. Pain referred from the neck is unaffected by movements of the shoulder but is aggravated by movement of the cervical spine.

X-ray examination

An antero-posterior film is sufficient for most conditions. An axial view, with the camera above the shoulder and the film in the axilla will give additional information. For the injured patient, who cannot easily move the shoulder, a trans-thoracic view is used and this is particularly valuable for demonstrating a posterior dislocation of the shoulder. An X-ray examination of the scapula must include a tangential view.

Treatment

Traumatic conditions

Fractures

For most fractures, analgesic tablets for 2–3 days and a triangular sling for the injured arm are all that is required. The attached muscles will draw the fractured clavicle or scapula back into anatomical alignment. Gravity will similarly correct most bony displacement at the upper end of the humerus. While the arm is in the sling it is important that the elbow be flexed above a right angle to prevent oedema forming in the hand and causing stiffness of the wrist and fingers. Fractures of the upper limb will be clinically united in three weeks in a child and usually in six weeks in an adult.

Dislocations

Shoulder.   An anterior dislocation, in which the head of the humerus moves medially to lie in a subcoracoid position, is by far the most common form of dislocation. In elderly subjects the dislocation can be reduced under Entonox, occasionally enhanced by 5–10 mg of intravenous diazepam. In young adults a general anaesthetic is required.

Kocher's manoeuvre, the preferred method of reduction, is performed in four stages. (1) With the elbow flexed to a right angle, pull down on the humerus against counter traction in the axilla. (2) Slowly externally rotate the arm to overcome the spasm in the subscapularis muscle. (3) Still applying traction and with the arm externally rotated to 90°, adduct the elbow across the patient's chest. (4) Relax the traction and internally rotate the arm to bring the fingers to lie on the opposite shoulder. Frequently the assistant, with hands clasped in the axilla, will detect movement of the humeral head back into the glenoid fossa during the second stage thereby making the remainder of the manoeuvre unnecessary. A high sling should be applied and a check X-ray taken. If the patient is under a general anaesthetic the check film should be taken before the patient wakes in case further manipulation is indicated.

Hippocrates manoeuvre, pulling on the extended arm against an assistant whose hands are placed in the axilla, should only be used if Kocher's manoeuvre has failed.

Posterior or the rare 'luxatio erecta' dislocations are usually easy to reduce by direct traction in the appropriate direction.

These manoeuvres are contraindicated when there is an associated fracture of the neck of the humerus or when the dislocation is more than 5 days old. Such patients should be referred directly to an orthopaedic surgeon.

Acromioclavicular and sternoclavicular dislocations. The former presents as a painful prominence at the point of the shoulder. The latter may be a retrosternal dislocation with a hollow beneath the skin at the sternoclavicular junction. This injury can damage major vessels. Conversely a prominence implies the clavicle has dislocated anteriorly. These patients should be prescribed analgesics and a sling and then be referred to an orthopaedic surgeon who will have the choice of either continuing the conservative treatment or operating to reduce the dislocation.

Rotator cuff injuries

The tendons of supraspinatus, infraspinatus and teres minor blend with the posterior part of the capsule of the shoulder joint and the subscapularis tendon reinforces the anterior part of the capsule. Together these structures form the 'rotator cuff'. Tears in the cuff result in localized tenderness and a painful limitation of movement of the shoulder joint. A serious tear of the supraspinatus may be repaired surgically in a young patient but most of the lesions respond to rest in a sling and analgesia. Diapulse is a valuable form of electrotherapy for reducing the pain and swelling of these injuries. After 2–3 weeks any localized residual pain may be eased by an injection of steroids into the painful area.

Non-traumatic conditions

Subacromial bursitis

The painful arc syndrome may or may not follow trauma as above and is characterized by rest pain, sleepless nights and reluctance to use the shoulder. It is treated by injecting steroids under the tip of the acromion and into the bursa. Analgesic tablets and a sling are advisable.

Supraspinatus tendinitis

This condition is extremely painful in the acute stage. The diagnosis is made by the radiological appearance of calcification in the supraspinatus tendon as it lies over the head of the humerus. Infiltration with steroids under the tip of the acromion usually brings quick relief. Diapulse therapy will also help to accelerate the cure. Only very rarely is it necessary to remove the tooth-paste-like material by curettage.

Pericapsulitis (periarthritis or the 'frozen shoulder')

A condition which inflicts pain and stiffness of the shoulder joint on patients over 50 years of age may arise following a fall or unaccustomed work such as painting a ceiling, or lying still in bed with an intravenous infusion in the arm, or it may arise spontaneously with no obvious cause. The characteristic features are the absence of gleno-humeral movement especially the total loss of external rotation. The pain is inflammatory in type and causes sleepless nights unless eased by anti-inflammatory drugs. Diapulse therapy is useful in reducing the pain. It can be supplemented by analgesics and a sling. Rest for the shoulder joint is important in the acute phase. When the pain is so diminished that sleep is no longer disturbed, the patient can begin gentle mobilization. The whole episode may last months and movement of the shoulder must not be forced to the point of provoking pain. The patient should be reassured that useful movement will return eventually.

Referred pain

Cervical spondylosis commonly presents with shoulder pain. Occasionally myocardial infarction, and rarely neuralgic amyotrophy and other neurological disorders may present with shoulder pain as a primary feature. Such patients have no objective signs in the shoulder.

Chapter 11

Injuries to the arm and elbow

Injuries to the arm and elbow can be divided into:

1. Fractures.
2. Dislocations.
3. Injuries to soft tissues.

If the injury is severe, complications due to damage to vessels or nerves must be detected and these will assume priority of importance over the bony injury. When the time comes to consider the radiological appearance one cannot assume that because there is now little displacement of the bones, other structures cannot have been damaged. At the moment of fracture or dislocation there was probably a wide discursion of the bony fragments with consequent tearing of the soft tissues. Normal elastic recoil and First Aid manoeuvres will have brought the fragments almost back into line by the time the X-ray is taken, but the soft tissue damage remains.

Fractures

Fractures of the shaft of the humerus

As with all limb fractures it is important to check for the integrity of the circulation and peripheral nerves: look for cyanosis or swelling of the forearm and hand; feel the radial pulse. In fractures of the middle third of the humerus check especially for damage to the radial nerve by asking the patient to extend the wrist and fingers. For fractures at the lower end of the humerus or dislocation of the elbow, inability to flex the index finger when 'making a fist' indicates damage to the median nerve; inability to abduct the fingers while they are in extension implies damage to the ulnar nerve. The median and ulnar nerve injuries will be confirmed by loss of sensation on the appropriate part of the palmar aspect of the hand and fingers. Radial nerve sensory innervation is very variable but when present it at least supplies the dorsum of the first web, between thumb and index.

Early manipulation of fractures of the shaft of the humerus is rarely necessary. If a collar and cuff sling is applied the weight of the arm gradually pulls the bony fragments into line. Plaster of Paris, if used, should only be applied as a slab on the outer aspect of the arm to protect it from further injury. A full arm cast is contraindicated; not only is it unnecessary but it adds the risk of circulatory occlusion if swelling occurs within the cast. After the initial treatment the patient is referred to an Orthopaedic Clinic for supervision until the fracture is healed in about 6 week's time.

Supracondylar fracture of the humerus

This is a childhood fracture resulting from a fall on the outstretched hand. The humerus breaks just above the condyles and the lower fragment is driven backwards stretching the brachial artery over the lower end of the upper fragment (*Figure 11.1*). This fracture is the most common cause of arterial occlusion in the upper limb, therefore always check the radial pulse before and after manipulation.

Manipulation, requiring an operator and an assistant, must always be performed under a general anaesthetic. The assistant

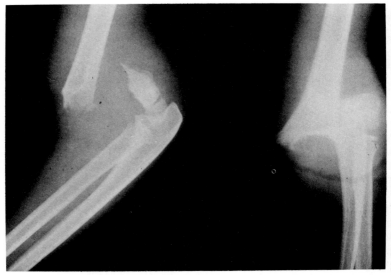

Figure 11.1 Supracondylar fracture of the humerus causing damage to the brachial artery

takes hold of the forearm and pulls distally with the elbow flexed at about 30°. If the lower end of the upper fragment has become impaled in the fibres of brachialis muscle it will be freed by this manoeuvre. It is then available to receive the lower fragment as this is pushed forward by the operator standing behind the elevated arm and using his thumbs to restore alignment.

After reduction the arm is fixed in a collar and cuff sling at an angle which does not occlude the radial pulse. There is still a risk of circulatory obstruction occurring due to swelling developing after the manipulation. Consequently, all these children should remain in hospital overnight for regular supervision of the circulation. If these precautionary steps are taken the feared complication of Volkmann's ischaemic contracture will be avoided.

Fracture of the lateral condyle of the humerus

This is a childhood fracture. Once the epicondyle and epiphysis of the capitulum have broken free the fragment usually rotates and cannot be reduced by closed manipulation. Also, accurate reconstitution of the articular surface of the elbow joint is so important that open reduction and fixation are usually required.

Fracture of the olecranon process of the ulna

This fracture is usually due to direct violence resulting in the proximal inch of the ulnar being broken off, the fracture line passing into the elbow joint. If the triceps expansion is still intact there will be minimal displacement and a triangular sling for 2 to 3 weeks is the only treatment required. More often the expansion is torn and the triceps tendon, which is inserted into the olecranon process, pulls the fragment of bone away from the rest of the ulna. Bony continuity can then only be restored by an open operation using a screw to re-position the fragment.

Fracture of the head or neck of the radius

This fracture is due to a fall on the outstretched hand and is seen in both children and adults. Force is transmitted up the forearm driving the head of the radius against the capitulum and either the outer portion of the head breaks off or the bone breaks just below the head across the neck. Pain and tenderness are felt on the lateral side of the elbow joint and movement is restricted and painful. If the standard X-ray views do not show a fracture, look for the 'fat-pad sign' (*see Figure 11.3*). If there is minimal displacement, or the fracture can be reduced by a closed manipulation, a collar and cuff sling is prescribed. If a closed reduction is impossible or unsuccessful, open reduction is indicated to prevent permanent impairment of elbow function.

Avulsed medial epicondyle of the humerus

This condition is not uncommon in children and is of little importance unless the epicondyle has been pulled into the elbow joint (*Figure 11.2*). If this occurs, manipulation under anaesthetic

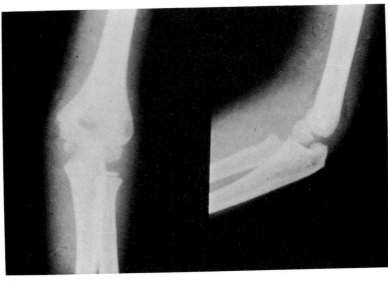

Figure 11.2 Avulsed medial epicondyle lying in the elbow joint

should be left to an orthopaedic surgeon who can proceed immediately to open operation and internal fixation if his manipulation is unsuccessful. Damage to the ulnar nerve may complicate this injury.

Interpretation of X-rays of the elbow

In the growing child, when the elbow region is 'full of epiphyses' it may be difficult to decide if a fracture is present. This dilemma is solved by taking an X-ray of the opposite, uninjured elbow which must be placed in the same degree of flexion and pronosupination to produce identical films for comparison.

Dislocations

Dislocation of the elbow joint

A patient with a recent dislocation of the elbow joint should have the dislocation reduced as quickly as possible before reactionary swelling makes the reduction more difficult. If, for one reason or another, the patient cannot be given a general anaesthetic within an hour of arriving at hospital then the manipulation should be performed under intravenous analgesia or Entonox.

Method of reduction

A surgeon and an assistant are required. The surgeon stands by the patient's shoulder, facing towards the patient's feet. He picks up the arm gently with both hands, the fingers encircle the arm gently above the elbow so that both thumbs rest on the tip of the olecranon process. Meanwhile, the assistant takes hold of the patient's wrist and pulls gently in the line of the deformity. Apart from exerting this gentle traction the assistant takes no other part in the manoeuvre. Pressing with his thumbs, the surgeon now pushes the olecranon over the curve of the trochlea and back into place. The gentle traction exerted by the assistant prevents the elbow flexing as the pressure is exerted by the surgeon and is an essential part of the manoeuvre. The arm is now immobilized in a collar and cuff sling, with the elbow in full flexion or as much flexion as is possible without occluding the radial artery. A check X-ray is taken to confirm the reduction and to display any associated fractures. The radial pulse must be carefully observed during the patient's stay in hospital and advice given to return immediately if the pain increases or the fingers change colour.

After treatment

It is important to explain to the patient that the elbow must remain at rest, in the sling for 3 weeks to give time for the injured tissues to heal. The patient can, and must, exercise his fingers but the elbow must remain immobilized. Plaster of Paris is not recommended because there is often considerable swelling after the reduction and a rigid cast could result in peripheral ischaemia.

After 3 weeks the swelling has subsided and the sling can be discarded. The patient is warned that full extension of the elbow will not return for some weeks or months; he can practise flexion exercises but any attempt to force extension will retard the progress. Physiotherapy cannot help, and passive exercises will only serve to hinder or prevent recovery. The patient should be seen at weekly intervals and, if it is found that he has lost full flexion, a further week's rest in a sling must be prescribed. The only consolation to offer the patient is that full or almost full movement will return eventually, provided myositis ossificans does not develop.

Pulled elbow

This condition is found in young children from the ages of about 1–3 years and is not uncommon. The child is brought by the mother with the complaint of pain in the arm and a refusal or reluctance to use it. There is often a typical history that the child has fallen and was rescued by the mother pulling him up by the affected arm. Examination of the limb shows no swelling and an X-ray shows no abnormality. It is believed that the lesion is caused by a subluxation of the head of the radius at the upper radio-ulnar joint.

Reduction of this subluxation is simple. One thumb is placed firmly on the head of the radius anteriorly. The forearm is held at the wrist and gently rotated through a full range while maintaining pressure over the radial head. As full rotation is reached, a click is felt by the thumb over the head of the radius. As soon as the child has recovered from the aggrieved surprise at this manoeuvre, a collar and cuff sling is applied, but this can be discarded after a few hours, the symptoms having disappeared.

Injuries to soft tissues

Traumatic effusion into the elbow joint

Many patients have elbow injuries which are less severe than those discussed so far. They may not come to hospital until 1 or 2 days after the accident. Their main complaint is of loss of movement rather than pain. It may be found on physical examination that they can only flex from 30° to 90° and pronosupination is also restricted. All these patients require X-ray. Fractures of the condyles of the humerus or the head of the radius may only be detected after careful scrutiny and study of a comparable X-ray of the opposite elbow. If no fracture is present there may still be an effusion into the joint. A useful guide to making this diagnosis is 'the fat-pad sign'. The pad of fat which normally lies flat on the anterior shaft of the humerus is raised like a pennant flag when there is an effusion in the joint (*Figure 11.3*). Such patients still require careful management. Myositis ossificans or fibrosis of the capsule may still occur if the joint is not adequately immobilized in the early stage. A collar and cuff sling is applied under the clothes, to keep the elbow at rest until the swelling and tenderness have disappeared. This may take 2 weeks and must be followed by the same careful regimen described above for dislocation of the elbow.

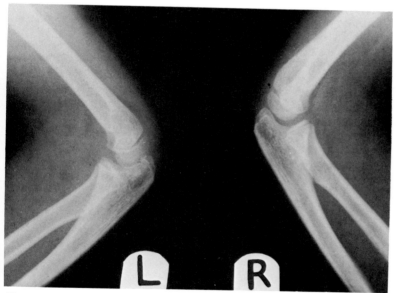

Figure 11.3 Positive fat-pad sign indicating an effusion into the left elbow joint. Note the dark shadows projecting anteriorly from the left humerus just proximal to the elbow joint (the right elbow is shown for comparison)

Many of these injuries occur in children and their parents are naturally anxious as to when they can return to school. There is no reason why they should not attend school with the arm in a sling. When the sling has been removed, the co-operation of the teacher should be enlisted to keep the child away from violent games or compulsory physical training; games should be avoided until full movement, or almost full movement is restored. If the elbow does not improve outside interference should be suspected.

Olecranon bursitis

Swelling of the olecranon bursa often follows a blow on the point of the elbow. Severe inflammatory changes can accompany the swelling so the condition can be divided into:

1. Inflammatory cases.
2. Non-inflammatory cases.

Inflammatory bursitis

The inflammatory swellings can vary from a tense red swelling with slight surrounding cellulitis, to a small, red swelling of the bursa surrounded by gross cellulitis with oedema reaching half-way down the forearm.

Treatment.   As with inflammatory prepatellar bursitis, conservative treatment is the most satisfactory. Incision into the inflamed bursa leaves a wound which is very slow to heal. If the swelling is very tense fluid should be assirated from the side of the swelling, not over the point of the elbow, using a wide-bore needle. If the fluid is purulent prescribe an antibiotic, otherwise treat with an anti-inflammatory agent. Rest in a sling; it may be several weeks before the induration around the bursa finally disappears.

Non-inflammatory bursitis

The non-inflammatory swellings of the bursa may follow a specific blow on the elbow, but can also follow recurrent irritation, e.g. beat elbow in miners.

Treatment.   If the swelling is very tense the fluid should be aspirated through normal skin at the side swelling. The swelling will probably recur within 2 to 3 days although, hopefully, not to the same degree, and the aspiration can be repeated. Firm bandaging and rest for the elbow discourages recurrence, but the bandaging is irksome and may be considered a greater disability than the original swelling. This condition will usually resolve spontaneously in time, but recurrent attacks causing inconvenience to the patient may be treated by excision of the bursa.

Chapter 12

Injuries to the forearm and wrist

History

Always ask the patient for his explanation of the symptoms. If there has been a recent injury, how did it happen? What is his normal occupation and has he recently been engaged in some unusual activity, e.g. home decorating, gardening or sport? Has the viability of the skin been jeopardized as when the limb is trapped between moving rollers? Is there a possibility of foreign material being buried in the wound? Was the wound self-inflicted?

Look

Inspect all aspects of the forearm and wrist and compare with the opposite side. Wounds will be obvious and fractures usually produce swelling or deformity. The common Colles' fracture results in a characteristic 'dinner fork' deformity of the wrist.

Feel

Ask the patient to indicate the site of the pain then support his forearm with one hand and gently palpate it with the other. Check the circulation and identify any areas of reduced sensation. Feel for crepitus either from a fracture or from an inflamed tendon sheath. Feel especially for tenderness in the anatomical snuff box which suggests a fracture of the scaphoid bone or the styloid process of the radius. Feel for foreign bodies buried under the skin.

Move

After recent injury movements are usually painful but it is important to confirm the integrity of the nerves and tendons. Extension of the fingers indicates that the radial nerve and its posterior interosseous branch are intact. Abduction and adduction of the extended fingers excludes damage to the motor branch of the ulnar nerve and abduction of the thumb, i.e. pointing the thumb to the ceiling when the hand is held flat, precludes motor damage to the median nerve. Abnormal findings should be correlated with sensory loss in the hand.

Tendon injuries will result in loss of movement in specific joints in the fingers or thumb or in the wrist. The divided ends of palmaris longus tendon may be seen in the wound; if this is the only injury the tendon does not merit repair. A patient who develops a spontaneous rupture of extensor pollicis longus tendon should be referred to a hand surgeon. This is an attrition rupture of the tendon which typically appears after a wrist injury or tenosynovitis and results in a drooping thumb.

X-ray

Fractures, dislocations and radioopaque foreign bodies will be demonstrated. Fractures of the scaphoid bone may be difficult to detect on the day of injury. Four views should be taken and a scaphoid cast applied even if no fracture is seen. When the cast is removed after 2 weeks the radiological examination should be repeated if the pain and tenderness is still present. By now resorption of the bone at the fracture line will make detection easier.

Treatment

Fractures

Undisplaced fractures

Protection and immobilization in a cast is necessary for 3 weeks in a child and 6 weeks in an adult.

Greenstick fractures

A buckle in the cortex at the end of a child's bone needs no manipulation. A greenstick fracture producing deformity in the mid-shaft of radius and ulna requires manipulation under an anaesthetic and immobilization in an above elbow cast. Minor degrees of deformity may be acceptable in a young child as they will be corrected by the subsequent growth of the bone.

Displaced fractures in the mid forearm

A fracture of the ulna may be satisfactorily manipulated and held in an above elbow cast. The radius can be more difficult because it is a curved bone and a fracture in the middle third may result in the two halves of the curve falling inwards towards the ulna. Manipulation should be performed by an orthopaedic surgeon adjacent to an operating theatre so that if closed manipulation fails open reduction can be performed.

Fractures of both radius and ulna in the mid forearm in a teenage or adult patient are notoriously unstable and often require open reduction and internal fixation.

Displaced lower third fracture in childhood

In a child the periosteum on the forearm bones is so thick and strong that 'periosteal splinting' makes it necessary to exaggerate the deformity almost to 90° before the fragments can be brought in line, but once they are hitched in place the situation is usually stable. This fracture must not be confused with the juvenile Colles' fracture.

Fractures at the lower end of the radius

The Colles' fracture is so common that detailed instructions for its management are given in Chapter 25. Do not confuse a Smith's fracture with a Colles' fracture. Smith's fracture is relatively unusual, the displaced fragment lies anteriorly and may be pressing on the median nerve. After reduction this fracture is often unstable; it may be necessary to immobilize the elbow as well as the wrist and to position the hand in supination.

Fracture separation of the lower radial epiphysis is a common childhood injury. Its precise reduction under a general anaesthetic is necessary to ensure subsequent normal growth. The manipulation is identical to that used for a Colles' fracture (see Chapter 25).

Fractures and dislocations in the carpus

Fracture of the scaphoid bone is a common injury and if the fracture line passes across the waist of the bone there is a possibility of avascular necrosis occurring in the proximal half of the bone. Similarly injury to the lunate may result in avascular necrosis (Keinboch's disease). Immobilization in a 'scaphoid cast' for 6 weeks from the day of injury is always advisable, the cast including the thumb up to the level of the interphalangeal joint.

Dislocation of the wrist is a rare injury requiring very considerable force. More frequently, although still rare, a dislocation occurs leaving only the lunate or the lunate and half the scaphoid still articulating with the lower end of the radius, or the lunate bone itself dislocates anteriorly. Lunar, perilunar or transcaphoid dislocations can be easily missed on X-ray. It is necessary to trace the outline of each carpal bone to ensure that there is no incongruous overlapping of one bone over another nor any abnormal gap between any of the carpal bones. These conditions all require urgent manipulation by an experienced surgeon and some require open reduction.

Sudek's atrophy

This is an abnormal vasomotor reaction which occasionally follows an injury to the wrist. The patient complains of a continuous throbbing pain which may persist for weeks or months. Such patients should be referred to a specialist surgeon for their subsequent management.

Plaster of Paris technique.   Important points in the use of plaster of Paris are listed in Chapter 25.

Soft tissue injuries around the wrist

Tenosynovitis

This commonly presents as an overuse syndrome with pain, swelling and crepitations on movement, at the back of the wrist. The precise structures involved vary. The radial wrist extensors are most commonly affected, but the extensor pollicis longus at Lister's tubercle, and the extensor digitorum communis at the distal border of the retinaculum may produce localized symptoms.

Rest in a splint or a plaster cast will usually abolish pain, and after a week or two the hand can be used again without discomfort. However, if the condition is occupational, it may well recur, and may even necessitate a change of job. If symptoms are not relieved by rest, local hydrocortisone injections are given. The tenosynovitis of the extensor pollicis must be treated with respect as it may be the precursor to eventual rupture, and surgical decompression is indicated if symptoms persist despite rest.

De Quervain's stenosing tenosynovitis

A particular form of tenosynovitis at the wrist described by De Quervain in 1895 requires special mention. It affects the sheath surrounding the abductor pollicis longus and extensor pollicis brevis tendons at the radial styloid.

The presenting features in A & E departments are often some form of injury, or overuse. The patient may well describe a blow on the wrist or a fall. There is pain radiating up the forearm and down into the thumb, exaggerated by movement and reproduced by hyperflexing the thumb. Tenderness is found accurately localized to the radial styloid, and sometimes there is a firm nodule at that site.

Steroid injections into the sheath relieve the pain, but for recurrent or longstanding cases surgical decompression of the sheath will be required.

Traumatic ganglion

Following minor trauma a tender, tense, cystic swelling develops in the region of the wrist joint. It is due to a herniation of the synovial membrane through the fibrous capsule of the joint. Initial treatment is by aspiration and bandaging, but, if the ganglion recurs, surgical excision usually brings a lasting cure.

Chapter 13

Hand injuries

The hand is the most frequently injured part of the body. Patients with hand injuries may form up to 10 per cent of the total case load of an Accident and Emergency Department. The importance for daily living of this complex, combined motor and sensory member is rarely appreciated until it is injured or mutilated. For most people, wage earning, running a home, and the majority of recreational pleasures depend on the integrity of their hands. Consequently, it is essential that every doctor working in an Accident Department be competent in the management of hand injuries. He must be able to make a comprehensive diagnosis, and understand clearly which conditions he may treat and which he should refer to a specialist hand surgeon.

After discussing the importance of the history and the physical examination, treatment of injuries to the various structures in the hand will be described. It is important to remember that these individual injuries do not necessarily occur in isolation and any one structure intimately affects another. The hand must be seen as an entity throughout the whole period of injury and rehabilitation.

History

The cause of the injury and the time at which it occurred must be noted. The nature of the trauma may suggest the possibility of foreign bodies being embedded in the wound or, as in the case of a hand trapped between moving rollers, that the damage to the skin and subcutaneous tissue will be much more extensive than is at first apparent. The reduction of a dislocated interphalangeal joint, performed on the sportsfield, is important to record because although physical signs may be minimal and the X-ray will be normal, there can be pain and stiffness for 2 to 3 weeks.

The circumstances in which the injury occurred are important, and should be recorded before they become embellished by frequent repetition. Industrial injuries may eventually result in medical evidence being required for litigation. Injuries sustained in the course of a crime may subsequently have to be described in a medicolegal statement or in a Court of Law, and if the details were not recorded at the time it will be impossible to recall them accurately at a later date. Self-inflicted injuries, serious though they may be, indicate that the patient has problems which go deeper than the physical wound and for which they are crying out for help.

Finally, this period of history-taking is invaluable for establishing rapport, for getting in touch with the patient. One must enquire as to which is the patient's dominant hand, and ask about his work, recreation and hobbies, and assess his attitude to his injury, because these factors may possibly influence the treatment and will definitely have a bearing on the success of the patient's rehabilitation.

Physical examination

This follows the classical steps of: look, feel, move and X-ray.

Look

Inspect the hand for bruising, swelling, deformity, inflammation and wounds, and examine both sides of the hand. Patients can be so perverse as to show a wound on the palmar surface and not think it necessary to mention that the extensor surface is also injured.

It will often be possible, by inspection alone, to diagnose a dislocated interphalangeal joint or, in a dangling finger, to suspect that the flexor tendons have been divided; but the patient still merits a full examination of the hand.

Feel

Approach the injured hand gently, just as one does when palpating the abdomen. Feel for tenderness, swelling, crepitus and sensory loss. To test for anaesthesia it is essential to obscure the patient's vision and, in the recently injured hand, it is preferable to stroke it lightly with your index finger or a piece or cotton wool rather than inflict further trauma by using a pin or needle.

Move

Movements are either 'active', which the patient performs himself, or 'passive' which you do to him. Always start with active movements first. Test the fingers for extension and flexion, including flexion of the distal interphalangeal joints. Ask the patient to spread the fingers in abduction. Examine the thumb for flexion, extension, adduction and abduction. Record any loss of full movement. Where there is loss of active movement, gently apply passive movement. If there is a fracture or dislocation, this will be difficult and painful. Conversely, if the deficit is due to nerve or tendon damage, passive movement will still be possible. There are some patients with severely crushed or mutilated hands in whom this precise distinction is not possible and they will require assessment by an experienced hand surgeon.

By this time it should be possible to form a definite opinion about damage to the major nerves:

1. *Radial nerve damage* above the elbow, causes a drop wrist and loss of extension of the fingers and a variable patch of anaesthesia centred over the dorsum of the first web.
2. *Ulnar nerve damage* causes paralysis of the intrinsic muscles of the hand, with a loss of abduction and adduction of the extended fingers. True opposition of thumb to index will also be absent. Anaesthesia usually involves the ulnar border of the palm, the little and half the ring fingers.
3. *High median nerve lesion,* in the region of the elbow: the patient cannot flex the index finger and has little or no flexion in the middle finger. He cannot abduct the thumb and has anaesthesia usually involving the palmar aspect of the radial 3½ digits.
4. *Low median nerve injury.* Division of the median nerve at the wrist is the most common of peripheral nerve injuries. It is caused by lacerations on a pane of glass or by self-inflicted knife wounds. The motor deficit from this injury is abduction of the thumb. To test for this the hand must be flat on the table, palmar side upwards, and the patient must attempt to point his thumb to the ceiling. All other movements in the fingers and thumb will be unaffected. The area of anaestheisa is the same as in the high median nerve lesion.
5. Injury to a digital nerve will result in anaesthesia on the side of the finger distal to the injury. The lesion should be repaired primarily.

Very occasionally when a patient has sustained a partial lesion of a nerve, the physical signs will be less precise.

X-ray

Antero-posterior and oblique views of the hand or a lateral view of a finger will reveal fractures or dislocation and any pre-existing abnormality of the bones or joints. Foreign bodies will usually be obvious. Metal stands out clearly, glass usually contains sufficient lead to make a definite shadow but plastic objects may be difficult to identify.

Treatment

Injuries to the skin and subcutaneous tissue

The principles of treatment are described in Chapter 18, and the management of the burned hand is discussed in Chapter 19. However, the hand poses certain problems because it is so frequently exposed to injury and these merit separate description.

Avulsed finger nail

If the nail has been completely ripped off, apply a non-adhesive dressing for a week to 10 days until the nail bed is re-epithelialized. Eventually a new nail will grow. If the nail has only been partially avulsed, leave it *in situ* as a protective biological dressing unless a nail bed injury is suspected, in which case the injury must be repaired. As the new nail grows it will expel the old one.

Sub-ungual haematoma

This is a common painful condition. The pain can be instantly relieved by trephining the nail with a hot wire to release the blood which is trapped beneath (*Figure 13.1*).

Local skin loss

When the wound edges cannot be brought together without tension, small partial thickness skin grafts can be taken from the thigh under a local anaesthetic, and used to cover the defect. Although they take well, as with all free grafts, they do not gain any sensory innervation. Often in the hand, bone, tendon or joint capsule are exposed in the wound and then a full thickness skin graft is required. If the area to be covered does not exceed 2 cm in any direction, a free graft can be taken from the forearm and the donor site closed by undermining the edges and performing a

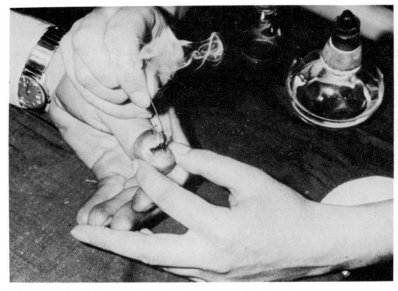

Figure 13.1 Trephining a sub-ungual haematoma of the thumb

primary suture. Donor and graft site should then be dressed and left undisturbed for 8 to 10 days. If the area to be covered is more than 2 cm across in any direction, then a skin flap is required and the junior doctor will be wise to seek advice of an experienced surgeon. Cross-finger flaps, thenar flaps, pectoral flaps, cross-arm flaps, inguinal flaps and neurovascular flaps may each be of value in appropriate circumstances.

Injuries involving rings

If the patient has a ring proximal to the injury it must be removed. If this is difficult and the skin is intact, soap may serve as a lubricant; failing this a ring cutter must be used (*Figure 13.2*). People working with machinery should not wear rings (*Figure 13.3*).

Traumatic amputations

Not involving the terminal phalanx

Apply a non-adhesive dressing–the finger tip will regenerate. If the cut is angled and there is extensive loss of the soft tissue, specialist advice should be sought.

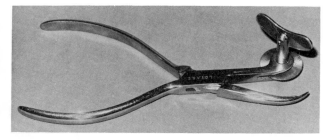

Figure 13.2 Ring cutter for removing rings from fingers

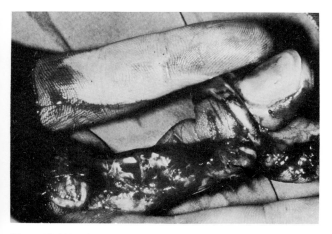

Figure 13.3 De-gloving of a finger resulting from a wedding ring caught in moving machinery

Involving the terminal phalanx

In the young child the finger can still be left to regenerate. In the older patient 'terminalization', in which the bone is nibbled back to allow primary skin closure without tension, is preferable. Admittedly this will result in a short finger, but it will have good sensation. For a patient such as a violinist, who requires a high degree of skill in his fingers, an expert surgical opinion should be obtained before any operation is performed.

Proximal to the terminal phalanx

The bone should be resected back to allow primary skin closure, making sure that the bone end is well covered by skin and subcutaneous tissue. Absorbable sutures should be used in finger-tips.

Re-implantation of severed digits

If the amputated portion of the digit has not been crushed, and particularly if more than one digit is involved, place the severed part dry in a plastic bag and lay the bag on ice. Then seek the advice of a hand surgeon.

In the thumb

The same principles apply, but it is more important to preserve the length of the thumb as well as sensation.

Post-operatively

In all these patients the hand should be rested in a high sling to discourage oedema formation. If the sutures are non-absorbable they should be removed after 7 to 10 days and then active rehabilitation begun immediately. Ideally the patient should be back at work within 4 to 6 weeks.

Tendon injuries

Extensor tendons

Three characteristic injuries occur in the extensor mechanism of the fingers:

1. Division of the tendon in a lacerated wound.
2. Middle slip rupture producing a boutonniere deformity.
3. Avulsion of the insertion of the tendon into the terminal phalanx producing a mallet finger deformity.

The divided tendon should be repaired using a figure-of-eight non-absorbable suture followed by immobilization of the wrist and finger in extension for 3 weeks. Immobilization may be achieved using either plaster of Paris or a foam padded malleable metal splint.

Middle slip rupture is not always easy to recognize when it first occurs but as the lateral slips of the extensor mechanism prolapse to the sides of the proximal interphalangeal joint, the typical 'boutonniere' deformity develops. The sooner surgical repair is performed the better will be the result.

Mallet finger deformity is a very common problem. Although various surgical procedures are in use it is doubtful if any of them produce better results than immobilizing the distal interphalangeal joint in a 'mallet finger splint' for 6 weeks (*Figure 13.4*).

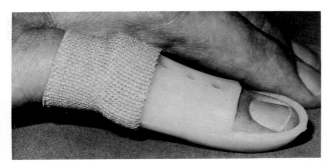

Figure 13.4 A plastic mallet finger splint used to immobilize the distal interphalangeal joint

Flexor tendons

The repair of these tendons is a task for an experienced hand surgeon. In the clean, incised wound, primary repair is indicated. In a contused or contaminated wound secondary repair is sometimes appropriate but in all cases expert advice is essential. Closed tendon injuries are often missed and they are especially amenable to primary repair. This is a typical rugby football injury.

Nerve injuries

Division of one of the main nerves, or one or more of the branches of the median or ulnar nerve in the hand or fingers, requires primary repair by a surgeon who is experienced in the use of an operating microscope.

Fractures

Metacarpals

Thumb. Because the first metacarpal is so mobile, when fractured it requires immobilization in plaster of Paris and, if this will not hold the fragments in a satisfactory position, internal fixation is indicated. Bennett's fracture involves the carpo-metacarpal joint with a free triangular fragment on the ulnar aspect. Treatment is either by a plaster of Paris forearm cast with moulding to extend the first metacarpal and allowing the distal two joints to flex, or by internal fixation.

Third and fourth metacarpals.   These are naturally splinted by the second and fifth metacarpals, so a light plaster of Paris cast or even a padded bandage is all that is necessary.

Second and fifth metacarpals.   Fractures of the shaft, if stable, are treated in a cast but internal fixation is more often required because of the mobility of these bones. Fracture of the neck of the fifth metacarpal is probably the most common fracture in the hand. It results from a blow delivered with a closed fist. If the angulation at the fracture exceeds 25° it should be manipulated under an anaesthetic. Then the ring and little fingers are immobilized round a roll of bandage with the metacarpopha-langeal joints held at 90° for 2 weeks.

Phalanges

If the fracture is displaced it requires reduction under either a local or general anaesthetic. Then for any phalangeal fracture the treatment depends on the position in which the fracture is stable. These are, in order or preference:

1. *Stable in any position* – apply neighbour strapping for 2 weeks.
2. *Stable in flexion* – strap the finger and the adjacent finger round a roll of bandage for 2 to 3 weeks.
3. *Stable in extension* – strap the finger to a malleable metal splint for 2 to 3 weeks.
4. *Unstable in any position* – internal fixation.

A compound, comminuted fracture of the terminal phalanx usually requires excision of the displaced fragments of the bone because they will not reunite and, if they are not removed, will result in a tender swollen finger end.

Injuries to joints

Direct trauma or dislocation of a finger joint will cause an effusion in the joint and swelling around it. A period of rest for 7 to 10 days should be followed by active exercises and wax baths. Diapulse therapy is of value in reducing the pain and swelling and thereby hastening recovery, and this can be applied daily through the dressing from the day of injury. A patient who only comes for treatment several days after the injury may develop a 'spindle finger' in which fibroblasts invade the swollen tissues and produce a characteristic chronic swelling which may take several months to resolve.

Rehabilitation

Active rehabilitation must be started immediately if any of the finger joints are stiff 10 days after skin repair, 3 weeks after tendon suture, or as soon as a fracture is stable. The only condition in which the earliest practical mobilization may be harmful is nerve suture. Traction applied too early to the suture line may produce scarring rather than nerve fibre regeneration.

Reference has already been made to the value of Diapulse therapy because it can be given during the period of immobilization. Wax baths and active exercises under the skilled supervision of a physiotherapist can be followed in a few days by group therapy in a hand class. Persistent stiffness or contractures may be treated by assisted exercises and corrective splinting. Occupational therapy is invaluable in preparing the patient to return to normal activities or, if this is not possible, enabling him to gain the maximum possible use from his hand.

Chapter 14

Injuries to the pelvis and hips

Patients with pelvic injuries fall into one of four categories:

1. Patients with generalized pelvic pain.
2. Patients with pain localized to a hip joint.
3. Patients with pain in the region of the sacrum and coccyx.
4. Patients with a limp or pain on walking.

Generalized pelvic pain

The pelvis is often injured in road traffic accidents. Pedestrians suffer a direct blow and car occupants, who are in a sitting position at the moment of impact, have the force transmitted up the thigh to be dissipated in the pelvis resulting in a fracture or dislocation or both. Such patients may only be able to give a vague history but the patient who is injured in the perineum from falling astride a hard object usually gives a graphic account of the accident.

Physical examination

The patient with a pelvic injury merits a full physical examination. The fractured pelvis can bleed so profusely as to cause oligaemic shock, especially in elderly subjects. Search for points of local tenderness around the pelvic bones and compress the pelvic ring from front to back and from side to side.

Examine the external urinary meatus for bleeding which implies damage to the urethra; examine the perineum for bruising and swelling; if the patient can urinate look for haematuria, if they cannot pass urine, urethral damage must be suspected.

Examine the abdomen for signs of visceral trauma (*see* Chapter 8).

Treatment

Severe bleeding from a fractured pelvis may be diminished by applying MAST (medical anti-shock trousers) while a blood transfusion is arranged.

Minor fractures of pubic or ischial rami or an isolated fracture of the wing of the ilium can be managed by bed rest at home if the domestic circumstances are suitable. However, many patients with fractures of the bony ring of the pelvis and all patients with damage to the urethra require in-patient management.

Pain centred on the hip joint

History

In the elderly patient, pain in the hip following direct or indirect violence, is strong presumptive evidence of a fracture. Patients may rest at home for several days hoping the pain will subside before they seek medical help.

Physical examination

A shortened limb lying in external rotation in an elderly patient suggests a fracture of the neck of the femur. Look for bruising and feel for tenderness around the greater trochanter and the neck of the femur. Movement of the hip may be limited and painful, but if the fracture is impacted there may be few signs and radiological examination will be necessary to establish the diagnosis.

X-ray examination

Good quality films are essential for an accurate diagnosis. The A-P film must include the whole pelvis and both hips to show possible fractures of the acetabulum, pubic or ischial rami, the femoral neck or trochanteric region. Some impacted fractures of the neck of the femur are at first only obvious on the lateral view but usually careful, repeated scrutiny of the bony trabeculae on the A-P film will confirm the diagnosis.

The neck of the femur is a common site for pathological fractures from secondary carcinoma. If this is suspected further physical and radiological examination may be necessary to locate the primary, for instance in bronchus, breast or prostate.

Treatment

Fractures

All patients with fractures of the neck or trochanteric region of the femur or of the acetabulum or adjacent rami of the pelvis require admission to hospital. No special splinting is required for their transport to the ward. However these elderly patients do deserve careful handling and must be kept warm all the time they are lying on a trolley.

Dislocations

Posterior dislocation of the hip is a relatively common injury. When it is associated with a more obvious fracture in the same limb it is all too easy to overlook, especially in the unconscious patient. The sciatic nerve may be damaged by the extruded head of the femur. It is wise to check its integrity by asking the patient to move the toes, before reducing the dislocation.

A general anaesthetic is required for the manipulation. The operator has to stand over the patient and apply traction to the thigh with hip and knee flexed to a right angle so as to draw the head of the femur forwards over the posterior lip of the acetabulum and back into the socket. It may be easiest to do this with the anaesthetized patient lying on a mattress on the floor. If the posterior rim of the acetabulum has been fractured, the loose fragment of bone may fall into the hollow of the acetabulum and so obstruct the reduction of the femoral head. This situation can only be remedied by an open reduction.

Anterior dislocation of the hip is a rare event. The patient arrives in great pain with the hip flexed and abducted. Reduction under anaesthetic must be done as soon as possible and the blood flow in the femoral vessels kept under close scrutiny.

Central dislocation of the hip. This follows a direct lateral blow commonly in a pedestrian hit by a vehicle, and the resulting disruption of the floor of the acetabulum with or without comminution of the pelvis may cause a life-threatening retroperitoneal haemorrhage.

Pain over the sacrum and coccyx

If the history reveals a fall onto the buttocks or a direct blow over the sacrum producing pain made worse by sitting, examination is directed to the sacrum and coccyx. Inspection may show swelling or bruising or both over this area. Palpation will reveal an area of acute tenderness within the area of general pain.

X-Ray examination may show a fracture of the body of the sacrum as one of several fractures in the pelvis. The lateral view may reveal a fracture, usually at the sacro-coccygeal junction, with angulation and a break in continuity, but frequently no fracture is evident.

Treatment

Patients with displaced or comminuted fractures of the body of the sacrum should be admitted for observation, especially because of the risk of visceral damage. If the fracture is limited to the coccyx, reduction is only necessary for patients with a gross deformity. Other patients are treated with analgesics, advised to use a soft cushion when sitting and to avoid constipation. With these precautions recovery can be expected in 2–3 weeks.

Pain on walking

A number of patients will attend complaining of pain in the hip or a limp, following a minor injury which occurred some days previously. These patients are frequently either old people or young children.

Elderly patients

Examination will reveal limitation of movement at the hip joint with pain at extremes of movement. Rarely, a stress fracture of the neck of the femur may be the cause of symptoms, but in the majority osteoarthrosis of the hip is present. If X-ray examination reveals a bony abnormality, the patient should be referred to the care of his general practitioner in the case of a chronic degenerative condition or admitted to hospital when a fracture or malignancy is demonstrated.

Children

Because there are many causes of a limp in children, such as an infected blister on the heel with lymphadenitis in the groin, every child merits a full examination, even though the history of trauma may be insignificant. In these days one should never find an undiagnosed congenital dislocation of the hip as the cause of a limp, or rather a waddling gait, in a toddler, but if such a tragedy is discovered it requires immediate referral for orthopaedic treatment. At a slightly older age of 4–10 years, avascular necrosis of the upper femoral epiphysis with fragmentation, and possibly later flattening of the epiphysis (Perthes' disease) is an important but uncommon cause which requires orthopaedic treatment.

Acute or chronic microbial infections of the hip joints are also fortunately now rare in Great Britain. They produce an ill child with an obvious systemic upset and usually an exquisitely painful hip, which will permit little or no movement.

'Transient synovitis' or 'the irritable hip', however, is a common condition. The physical signs of a synovitis of the hip are a painful joint with a reduced range of movement. A flexion deformity is the most characteristic single sign. To discover it the child should be lying flat on his back and the sound limb flexed to its fullest extent up to the abdominal wall. When a flexion deformity is present the thigh of the affected limb will be spontaneously raised off the couch and cannot be made to lie flat again. The hip may, however, appear normal, but on attempted movement spasm is encountered which prevents full excursion of the joint. It is advisable to admit any child who exhibits such a sign for observation and possible further investigation. If physical and radiological examinations are both negative the mother can be reassured and asked to bring the child back if the symptoms have not completely disappeared in 4–5 days. A normal erythrocyte sedimentation rate is helpful in reaching the decision.

One other important orthopaedic condition which often presents at the A & E department is that of slipped upper femoral epiphysis. This disorder more than any other illustrates the fact that disease in the hip may present as pain in the knee. Consequently any child between the ages of 9 and 14 years complaining of spontaneous onset of a vague pain around the knee should have his hips examined. Limitation of movement in the hip indicates the necessity for radiological examination and urgent orthopaedic advice should be sought for any patient who has asymmetrical upper femoral epiphyses.

Chapter 15

Injuries to the thigh and knee

The knee joint is a gracious joint. If you take time to find out the precise details of the accident and pay the joint the compliment of a thorough physical examination, it will yield up most of its secrets and the diagnosis will become clear. Every injured knee joint must be examined in a comprehensive and systematic manner. To do this the patient must have his trousers removed or her skirt pulled up and tights removed and be lying on his/her back on a couch with good overhead illumination. The examination has four consecutive stages: look, feel, move and X-ray. By the time the third stage is completed the radiological findings of the fourth stage will often be predictable or, indeed, an X-ray examination may have become unnecessary.

History

There are four basic questions to ask:

1. How long is it since the injury occurred?
2. What was the exact nature of the injury?
3. How have the symptoms evolved since the accident happened?
4. Are there any other local or general medical factors which might be relevant?

How long?

Unless prevented by exceptional circumstances, a patient with a fracture or a serious injury to a ligament or tendon around the knee joint comes to hospital within 24 hours of the accident occurring. Patients who wait more than a day before seeking medical aid either have a mild effusion which is taking time to resolve, or they had previous pathology in or around the knee joint which has been aggravated or 'brought to light' by the injury.

What exactly happened?

A direct blow on the patella from a fall on the point of the knee, or crushing the knee against the dashboard of a car in a road traffic accident, will produce a fracture of the patella. In the car accident the force may also have been transmitted up to the hip joint producing a fracture or dislocation or both, so when the leg is injured in a car accident always examine the hips as well.

A blow from the bumper of a car hitting the outside of a pedestrian's leg may produce an impacted, depressed fracture of the lateral condyle of the tibia.

A twisting injury, in which the foot remains fixed to the ground and the body swings round, is the classic method of producing a torn meniscus.

The elderly person who stumbles over a raised paving stone, falls to the ground and then cannot fully extend the knee, will have ruptured the quadriceps tendon.

What happened next?

Was it possible to continue working for a while or to continue playing after the accident occurred? Did the swelling come on immediately – probably haemarthrosis – or did it come on slowly over the next few hours – most likely a serous effusion.

Was it possible to extend the knee fully after the accident? Has there been 'locking' of the knee? This is a very useful item of information provided the patient fully understands what is meant. 'Surgical locking', implying a torn meniscus, means that the patient can extend the knee to a certain point and then no further. The loss of full extension may be only 5° but it is definite and consistent. The doctor must always be sure that the patient's description of 'locking' conforms with this definition.

Other relevant medical history

The child at puberty, especially an overweight or over-athletic boy, may have a traction apophysitis of the tibial apophysis (Osgood-Schlatter's disease). A patient with a bleeding diathesis may have a spontaneous haemarthrosis. Most common of all is the patient with osteoarthritis of the knee joint. Such patients have managed fairly well until some relatively trivial injury aggravates their previously mild symptoms and makes them seek medical help.

Physical examination

Look

Stand back and look at the knee in good light, comparing it with the opposite knee. The swelling or deformity from a fracture of femur or tibia may be obvious. Dislocation of the patella, most common in young women, presents as a rigid, painful knee with a lump on the lateral side. When the patella tendon is torn – a young person's injury – the patella lies higher than on the other side. When the quadriceps tendon is torn – an old person's injury – there is the characteristic gap or hollow an inch above the patella. Dislocation of the knee – a rare but disastrous injury – presents with the leg no longer in line with the thigh and one's first concern must be for the circulation below the knee.

Fluid or inflammation in the bursae around the knee joint will be seen as localized swellings – pre-patella or infra-patella or behind the knee on the medial side – a semi-membranosus bursa. Effusion into the knee joint itself shows first of all by filling out the para-patella fossae – the hollows that normally lie on each side of the knee cap (*Figure 15.1*). Then the supra-patella bursa will fill and finally the whole joint may be bulging with a tense effusion of 100 ml or more.

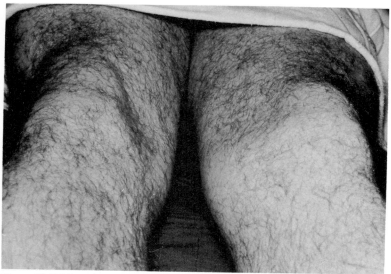

Figure 15.1 This patient shows a normal para-patella fossa on the right but the left knee has a slight effusion and the fossa has filled out

Feel

First of all check the circulation in the limb, if necessary by palpation of the posterior tibial and dorsalis pedis arteries; then seek to localize the tenderness. A torn meniscus produces tenderness precisely along the joint line in the sulcus between femur and tibia on the appropriate side. A partially torn collateral ligament produces a more diffuse tenderness reaching up to the femoral condyle.

In the presence of a large effusion there will be a 'patella tap'. The patella is being held off the femoral condyles by the fluid in the joint; pressing on it depresses it a few millimetres until it impinges on the femur. A dislocated patella will be palpable on the lateral side of the joint. A fractured patella will be covered by bruising and oedema and it may be possible to elicit crepitus as bony fragments are palpated. A torn patella tendon results in a high riding patella with a hollow distal to it, and a ruptured quadriceps tendon leaves a soggy hollow just proximal to the patella.

Swellings limited to individual bursae will be palpable and the area will be warm and tender if there is active inflammation.

Localized hard lumps around the joint may be due to loose bodies, which will move as they are palpated; osteophytes which do not move; or, on the lateral aspect below the joint line, a cyst of the lateral cartilage. Small mobile loose bodies in the pre-patella bursa may be palpated; they give rise to pain on kneeling and may require surgical removal.

Move

As with all joints, the movements are either active or passive. Examine the range of active movements first. Can the patient fully extend the knee? How far can he flex it compared with the opposite knee? Finally can he lift the heel off the couch without bending the knee – a test for the integrity of the extensor mechanism.

Passive movements are used to assess the integrity of the ligaments and the menisci. To examine the medial collateral ligament of the knee joint flex the knee 10–15°, take hold of the ankle from the medial side with one hand, then place the other hand over the lateral aspect of the knee joint. Now apply a 'valgus strain' – trying to move the ankle away from the midline while holding the knee still with the other hand. One of three things will happen:

1. There will be no movement and the patient will not complain – the medial collateral ligament is intact.
2. There will be movement and pain. When you relax the strain, the leg will spring back into line and you will feel the impact as femoral and tibial condyles come back into contact. This is referred to as 'springing' of the joint – there is an incomplete tear of the medial collateral ligament.
3. In the presence of a complete tear the joint opens widely – this should be confirmed by X-ray.

Now reverse the position of the hands and test the lateral collateral ligament (*Figure 15.2*).

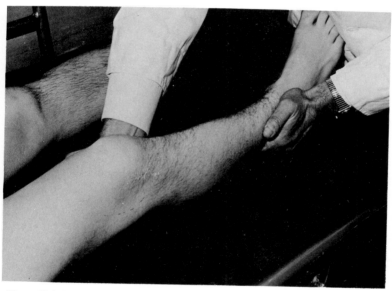

Figure 15.2 Applying a varus strain to the knee joint to test the integrity of the lateral collateral ligament

Next, examine the cruciate ligaments. With the knee flexed to 90° take hold of the leg with both hands just below the knee and attempt to rock the tibia forwards and backwards. If the cruciates are torn there may be abnormal movement (drawer sign) unless there is a large effusion which, by tightening the capsule, prevents the movement.

Finally, perform McMurray's manoeuvre to elicit the click of a torn cartilage. Stand beside the knee, place the upper hand over the front of the knee joint, fingers on one side, thumb on the other. Take hold of the dorsum of the foot with the other hand. Flex the knee as far as it will go, then rotate the tibia on the femur, first one way and extend the knee then, after re-applying flexion, rotate the tibia the other way and extend the knee. A click, heard or felt, during this manoeuvre, coupled with the tenderness along the joint line indicates a torn meniscus. Unfortunately, within an hour or two of injury there may be such a large effusion in the joint that this manoeuvre is not possible. The effusion must be treated and the test applied when the swelling has subsided in about a week's time. If complete rupture of ligaments is suspected, a stress view under analgesia (e.g. Entonox) should be done by the doctor.

X-Ray

Antero-posterior and lateral views will show fractures or dislocations, changes due to osteoarthrosis or other local pathology in the bones around the joint. Loose bodies due to osteochondritis dissecans may be seen but to demonstrate the defect in the femoral condyle, from which they have come, a 'tunnel view' through the intercondylar notch is usually necessary. A fabella, a sesamoid bone in the lateral head of gastrocnemius (*Figure 15.3*). must not be confused with a loose body.

Careful scrutiny of the cortical line of each bone should reveal any fractures. The head and neck of the fibula should be included in the film and they merit special attention because of the close association of the lateral popliteal nerve with the neck of the fibula and the attachment of the lateral collateral ligament of the knee joint to the head of the fibula. Most fractures around the knee are so gross as to be obvious at first glance but a fracture of one of the tibial spines, to which the cruciate ligaments are attached, may be missed if the upper surface of the tibia is not examined carefully.

Treatment

If the circulation is impaired, steps to restore it by manipulation or open operation take precedence over all other local considerations.

Fractures of the femur

These are treated by the application of a Thomas splint. If the procedure is painful, we strongly recommend the use of Entonox (50 per cent nitrous oxide and 50 per cent oxygen) to allow an approximate reduction of the fracture and the application of the

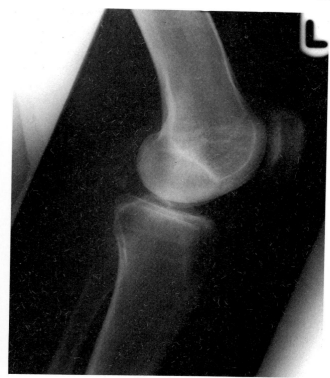

Figure 15.3 A fabella is a sesamoid bone in the head of the gastrocnemius (not to be confused with a loose body)

splint. An alternative method of providing analgesia is to perform a femoral nerve block. Check the circulation again after putting on the splint. The patient is then admitted to the orthopaedic ward.

Fractures of the upper end of tibia and fibula

These are usually treated with a long leg plaster of Paris cast but a depressed fracture of the lateral tibial condyle may require open reduction and internal fixation.

Dislocation of the knee

This should be reduced as quickly as possible using Entonox or a general anaesthetic because of the risk to the circulation. The patient will then be admitted to the orthopaedic ward with his leg in a Thomas splint.

Dislocated patella

It may be possible to reduce the dislocation by pressure on the outer side of the patella as the leg is extended. If this proves too painful, Entonox will allow an easy reduction. A compression bandage should be applied, crutches prescribed, and the patient referred to the Fracture Clinic.

Fracture of the patella

If the patient can lift the heel off the couch with the knee extended, then the extensor aponeurosis must still be intact despite the fracture of the patella and an ankle-to-groin plaster of Paris cylinder should be applied and the patient referred to the Fracture Clinic. Otherwise the patient must be admitted to hospital for reconstruction or excision of the patella.

Tendinous and ligamentous tears

Partial tears of the collateral ligaments should be treated by a compression bandage for 5–7 days, followed by a plaster of Paris cylinder when the swelling has subsided. If the swelling is small, at the time of the initial visit the plaster cylinder can be applied immediately and worn for 2–3 weeks. The complete tear should be referred to an orthopaedic surgeon with a view to surgical reconstruction. Tears of the patella tendon or the quadriceps tendon also require admission to hospital for surgical repair.

Torn meniscus

A twisting injury, followed by swelling of the knee joint and tenderness over the cartilage suggests a meniscus injury. Some patients come in considerable pain with the knee locked in about 60° of flexion. A general anaesthetic is required to allow manipulation to unlock the knee, otherwise a compression bandage is applied and the patient given crutches and referred for definitive treatment when the effusion has subsided.

Traction apophysitis (Osgood-Schlatter's disease)

Occasionally children, usually boys, between the ages of 10 and 15 years limp into the Emergency Department. They are found to have a swollen, tender area over the tibial tubercle at the insertion of quadriceps tendon. Usually a supporting bandage and instructions to avoid cycling and football are all that is required. For the more refractory causes a plaster of Paris cylinder for 1 to 2 months may be necessary.

Stress fracture

Another result of overuse is a stress fracture usually of the upper end of the tibia. The onset of symptoms is gradual and there is local tenderness and swelling. An X-ray will confirm the diagnosis.

Traumatic synovitis

The number of patients with this diagnosis will probably equal or surpass the total of all other patients with injuries around the knee joint. This is because the knee responds to any moderate trauma by forming a serous effusion in the joint. This is frequently seen in the knee which has early arthritic changes. The knee is generally tender and movements are restricted. Occasionally the effusion is so large that the knee is bulging and the patient is in considerable pain. This situation justifies aspiration of the joint. After full surgical preparation, with an aseptic technique, fluid is aspirated through a needle introduced on the lateral aspect of the joint under the upper half of the patella. The aspirate may contain globules of fat, indicating that there is a fracture involving the knee joint, or it may contain blood – a haemarthrosis. After the aspiration, or immediately if aspiration is not necessary, the knee joint must be immobilized.

Tone in the quadriceps muscle should be maintained by teaching the patient to do 'static exercises', that is tightening and relaxing the muscle within the bandage or plaster cast for, say, 5 minutes every 3 hours. Cast or bandage should be removed after a week and replaced with an elasticated support, such as Tubigrip, and the patient can start walking, with the aid of crutches or a stick if necessary. If they have not kept up the tone in the quadriceps muscle the patients may complain of the knee 'giving way' as they walk. This complaint, together with pain and a chronic effusion, will only disappear when muscle power returns to normal.

Bursitis

Either the pre-patellar or the infra-patellar bursa may become swollen or inflamed. Usually this follows repetitive minor trauma and it may be complicated by bacterial infection. Incision is not recommended as the surgical wound is often slow to heal.

Aspiration will relieve the pain and give a sample of fluid for bacteriological study. A compression bandage, rest, anti-inflammatory drugs, and if necessary antibiotic therapy should produce a cure within a week to 10 days. The patient must then take care to protect the knee or avoid the trauma which precipitated the acute episode.

Myositis ossificans

Although this condition may develop following trauma around the elbow joint it is seen most frequently in the thigh. The usual story is of a blow on the thigh during a football game. After the game the thigh becomes increasingly painful and flexion of the joint aggravates the pain. Over the next few days a firm swelling, some 10–15 cm in diameter, develops in the thigh. Massage or exercises only serve to aggravate the symptoms. The patient comes to the Accident Department complaining of the painful swelling and a range of flexion of less than 90°. The typical history with these findings on physical examination gives the clinical diagnosis of myositis ossificans. The substantive diagnosis is made by X-ray examination (*Figure 15.4*). The radiological evidence, an area of hazy calcification lying anterior to the femoral shaft, is not seen for at least 10 days after the injury and may not appear for 6 weeks. Treatment, therefore, should be started on the clinical diagnosis alone and X-rays taken at weekly intervals to check for the appearance of a calcified shadow and then to document its progress.

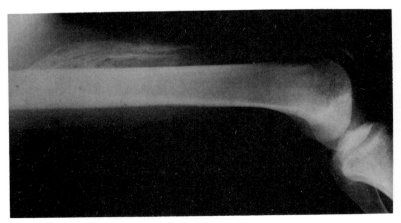

Figure 15.4 Myositis ossificans in the thigh

Treatment consists of stopping all massage or exercises and putting the thigh at rest by applying a plaster of Paris cylinder. This immobilization should continue for 6 weeks or until all local tenderness in the thigh has gone, whichever is the longer. Thereafter, gradual knee exercises can be started under physiotherapy surpervision. Any recurrence of pain in the thigh at this time indicates the need for a further 3 weeks' immobilization. By this time the X-ray appearance may show a dense, bone-like shadow in the thigh, but once the edges of the shadow are smooth and well defined the condition will not grow any further and the patient can hope to return to a full range of sporting activity.

Chapter 16

Injuries to the leg and ankle

These common injuries will be described under three headings:

1. Injuries to the bones.
2. Injuries to muscles.
3. Injuries to tendons and ligaments.

Injuries to bones

All open fractures must be admitted to hospital under the care of an orthopaedic surgeon. In the Emergency Department the doctor must check the circulation distal to the fracture. If the circulation is impaired an immediate manipulation under Entonox is indicated, not to reduce the fracture, but to take the pressure off the vessels. A sterile dressing and a temporary padded splint are then applied and the patient given an analgesic injection. It is important to make sure that there is no central trauma to head, thorax or abdomen, which could threaten life, before turning all one's attention to the peripheral injury. Also, remember that the limb may be injured at more than one level. Fractures or dislocations of the hip can easily be overlooked because of a fracture of the leg which is more obvious and more painful.

Closed fractures will be treated initially either by the emergency doctor or by the orthopaedic staff according to local arrangements and depending on the severity of the injury. Fractures of the tibia and fibula, if displaced, will be reduced under a general anaesthetic and then, as with undisplaced fractures, immobilized in an above-knee plaster of Paris cast (*see* Chapter 25). Only if the fracture affects one malleolus only, and the fracture line is distal to the level of the main tibio-talar articular surface, should a below-knee plaster cast be used.

All these plaster of Paris casts must be padded, and the patient must not bear weight on them for at least the first 24 hours. The circulation in the toes must be checked after 24 hours, the patient having been instructed to seek medical advice earlier if the toes become swollen or blue.

Injuries to muscles

Anterior compartment syndrome

This patient complains of pain down the front of the leg aggravated by walking or running. The syndrome is seen most frequently in people who have made an extraordinary muscular effort or in an athlete who has just started training. Presumably there has been a partial muscle tear of the dorsiflexor muscles with bleeding in the closely confined compartment between tibia and fibula. Resting the leg as much as possible and Diapulse therapy to dissipate the oedema will relieve the symptoms.

Injury to the calf muscles

Following a sudden muscular effort, such as running to catch a bus, a patient complains of pain in the calf. Palpation will reveal a localized area of tenderness due to rupture of some of the fibres of the gastrocnemius muscle. Treatment is to have a 2–2.5 cm raise on the heel of both shoes for a couple of weeks.

Injuries to tendons and ligaments

Ruptured Achilles tendon

This condition is seen in middle-aged people, especially if they are overweight. A common cause is the so-called 'keep-fit' class. A complete tear is such a dramatic event that the patients look round to see who hit them. Then, finding that they can no longer rise onto their toes but only shuffle along flat-footed, they usually make the diagnosis themselves. Treatment is by surgical repair.

A partial tear of the tendon presents as a painful swelling behind and above the heel, but without the characteristic gap that occurs when the tendon is completely torn. The patient can still plantar flex the foot against resistance, but it is painful to do so. Treatment is to apply a below-knee plaster of Paris cast with the ankle in equinus to rest the tendon, and crutches are provided. This is the only situation in which the foot should be immobilized in plantar flexion. The patient is then referred to an orthopaedic surgeon for subsequent management.

The recent surge of enthusiasm for 'jogging', particularly amongst middle-aged men, many of whom are seeking rehabilitation after a coronary thrombosis, has resulted in an increase in the number of patients with partial tears and strains of the calf muscles or tendons.

Sprained ankle

This extremely common condition falls into three categories: the minor injury, the severe, and a broad intermediate group.

Minor injury

Most people who sustain a minor sprain look after it themselves but a few come to hospital. They walk in with little or no limp and the swelling and tenderness are minimal. They need reassurance, advice and perhaps a crepe bandage.

Severe injury

These are patients in whom the stability of the ankle joint is at risk or disrupted. Their lesion is extremely painful, they cannot bear weight on the foot, there is gross swelling and tenderness. An X-ray of the ankle may show fractures of medial or lateral malleoli or both, the fracture line being sufficiently high in the malleolus to remove one of the buttresses of the ankle mortice. If no bony injury is shown on X-ray, films taken with the foot stressed into maximum inversion, then maximum eversion will show if there is abnormal movement of the talus within the ankle mortice due to complete rupture of medial or lateral ligaments. To perform this investigation adequately in the acute stage may require the use of Entonox or intravenous analgesia. If the sprain, or rupture, involves the medial, deltoid ligament surgical repair is recommended. If only the lateral ligament is involved, opinions vary as to whether surgical repair or plaster of Paris immobilization is indicated in this situation. The emergency doctor should consult his orthopaedic colleague.

Moderate injury

These patients are often incapacitated by their injury, even though the integrity of the ankle joint is not in doubt. They provide a substantial part of the work of the A & E department. An inversion injury, producing a sprain or partial tear of the lateral ligament of the ankle is the most common. Because the medial ligament is stronger than the lateral it is not sprained so easily but, when it is, it implies that there has been a considerable amount of force involved in the accident and an X-ray examination is advisable.

The lateral ligament has its origin at the lower end of the fibula, or lateral malleolus and it fans out with three distinct bands. The talo-fibular ligament is sprained when the inversion injury occurs with the ankle fully plantar flexed as in the take-off position when running. The pain, swelling and tenderness are then above and anterior to the lateral malleolus. Pain and swelling immediately below the lateral malleolus implies that the fibulo-cuboid ligament has been sprained, which occurs when the inversion injury takes place with the foot in the neutral position. The fibulo-calcaneal ligament is rarely torn in isolation. Careful examination, to localize the area of maximum tenderness, coupled with knowledge of the local anatomy will result in a precise diagnosis.

The tip of either malleolus may be fractured off in this type of injury. If there was an element of rotation in the force applied to the ankle, the lateral malleolus may be fractured obliquely. This fracture line is often invisible on the antero-posterior film, and will only be seen following careful scrutiny of the lateral film because the medial malleolus and talus are in the same line of projection.

The same type of inversion injury may produce a fracture of the base of the fifth metatarsal due to the pull of peroneus brevis tendon in its attempt to take the whole weight of the body, or an avulsion of a small fragment from the cuboid attachment of the calcaneo-cuboid ligament. On palpation of these bony points it may be possible to decide that there is no bony injury present. If one can state this with confidence, then no X-ray is necessary. If there is any doubt at all, take an X-ray of the ankle to show the malleoli, and an X-ray of the foot to show the fifth metatarsal. Reviewing these patients has shown us that the incidence of fractures associated with sprained ankles is four times greater in patients over 50 years of age than in younger patients.

If a fracture is demonstrated on X-ray then a below-knee plaster of Paris cast is applied and the patient referred to the Fracture Clinic.

If there is no fracture, the intensity with which the lesion is treated depends on the urgency with which the patient wishes to return to full activity. If there is no great urgency then adhesive strapping is applied from toes to calf. The patient is advised to rest the ankle for 24 to 48 hours and then gradually to resume walking.

After a week to 10 days when the strapping is removed, the symptoms are usually greatly improved. A crepe bandage or Tubigrip dressing may be required for a further week.

For the patient for whom two weeks is too long a period of reduced activity, physiotherapy can speed recovery. Diapulse therapy will disperse the oedema and thereby reduce the pain. If this is followed by supportive bandaging and supervised walking exercises, treatment on three successive days will relieve most of the symptoms. A double blind trial using Diapulse therapy showed that on average 80 per cent of symptoms were relieved after 3 days of treatment*.

* Wilson, D. H. (1971). *British Medical Journal*, **2,** 269

Chapter 17

Injuries to the foot

Patients coming to the Accident and Emergency Department with foot problems fall into one of two groups:

1. Those who have sustained a specific, recent injury.
2. Those with pain in the foot of recent onset, whose symptoms are attributed to some recent imprecise minor injury.

Physical examination of a recently injured foot will elict pain and swelling, but it is not usually possible to make a definite diagnosis without X-ray examination. Because patients wish to walk on their feet, that is to transmit their whole body weight through each foot in turn, it is important to know if the bony structures are intact and this necessitates a radiological examination. Emergency management of the more common injuries of the foot are as described below.

Group 1 – a recent specific injury

Fractures of the calcaneum

This fracture results from a fall from a height onto the heels. The patient is carried into hospital with a painful swollen heel. It is essential to remember that the force of the fall may well have been transmitted up the leg to the hip and spine producing fractures at either or both of these levels, even though the patient does not immediately complain of them.

If the fracture involves the subtalar joint and there is extensive swelling, the patient should be admitted to hospital for elevation of the foot and early exercises, in order to minimize, so far as possible, the long-term complications of stiffness and pain in the foot.

For fractures not involving the talo-calcaneal joint a well padded below-knee plaster of Paris cast or a wool and crepe dressing is applied and the patient referred to the Fracture Clinic. Patients with fractures of both os calcis may require admission to hospital for social reasons.

Fracture of the talus

This fortunately rare injury should always receive early expert orthopaedic treatment because of:

1. The risks of necrosis of the skin if there is a dislocation associated with the fracture.
2. Avascular necrosis of the head of the talus.

Mid-tarsal dislocation

This injury produces a very painful swollen foot. A junior doctor examining the X-ray may fail to appreciate the seriousness of the injury because there is no fracture. Examining the radiological appearance of each individual bone is necessary but one must also study the relationship of each bone with its neighbours. In this condition the proximal articular surface of the navicular is no longer articulating with the head of the talus, and a reduction under anaesthetic is required. The sooner the manipulation is attempted, the easier it is: delay allows oedema to develop and makes the reduction more difficult. Following the reduction a well padded plaster cast is applied and the patient instructed to elevate the foot, and sleep with it on a pillow for the next 48 hours. Admission to hospital may be necessary after the reduction in order to supervise the circulation. A bipartite or accessory navicular bone must not be mis-diagnosed as a fracture of the navicular; it is recognizable by its smooth, rounded, clearly defined edges.

Fractures of the metatarsals

Fracture of the base of the fifth metatarsal is discussed in Chapter 16 under 'Sprained ankles'. Fractures of the shafts of the metatarsals do not usually need any manipulation; a padded below-knee plaster of Paris cast is the appropriate treatment.

Fractures of the necks of the metatarsals often occur in the guise of a 'March fracture'. After a long hike in heavy footwear the patient complains of pain and tenderness in the region of the necks of the second or third metatarsals. At this stage an X-ray may fail to show a fracture. Elastoplast strapping from toes to calf will give sufficient support. If the symptoms are still present after 2 weeks a second X-ray may show bone resorption at the site of the fracture with a small amount of callus around it. This is a 'March fracture'. Some patients may need a walking cast for as long as 6 weeks.

Fracture of the toes

The hallux

Crushing injuries of the big toe are very common in areas of heavy industry. Protective footwear with steel toe caps should make the injury a rarity, but this has yet to happen. Manipulation of the fractured phalanges is rarely necessary and treatment is directed towards protecting the toe until the tenderness disappears and healing is well advanced. This is done by applying a plaster of Paris slab or a collodion splint over the toe and, if necessary, applying a pad of orthopaedic felt under the heads of the metatarsals. With this treatment most patients can return to work within a couple of weeks.

The smaller toes

Displacement requiring manipulation is rare. Simple immobilization by strapping the injured toe to its uninjured neighbour for 1 to 2 weeks is all that is necessary. Painting gentian violet 1:200 between toes before applying the strapping discourages an exacerbation of the all too common 'athlete's foot'.

The treatment of the bruised smaller toes without a fracture is exactly the same and it is doubtful, therefore, if X-ray examination of an injured smaller toe is necessary.

Injured feet in small children

The young child is not able to localize accurately a pain in the leg. He limps in, or is carried in, and complains of a pain in the foot. It is wise to examine the leg as well as the foot, because an undisplaced spiral fracture of the tibia may well present in this way.

Group 2 – no recent specific injury

'Osteochondritis'

In children and adolescents, avascular necrosis of the navicular bone (Kohler's disease), or a similar osteochondritis of the heads of the second or third metatarsals (Freiberg's disease)–this latter condition being more common in young adults–may produce pain in the foot. On X-ray the navicular looks dense and small, the metatarsal heads are broad and flat with a thickened neck. The symptoms usually respond to supportive bandaging. Only occasionally is surgical treatment necessary. Traction apophysitis of the os calcis (Sever's disease) is another example of an overuse syndrome.

Metatarsalgia

Pain across the metatarsal joints is a common condition in older people probably due to being overweight and having poor tone in the intrinsic muscles of the foot. 'Emergency treatment', if this is ever necessary, consists of applying a metatarsal pad under the metatarsal heads and referring the patient for an orthopaedic opinion. Morton's metatarsalgia is a specific condition due to a digital neuroma.

Hallux rigidus

While out walking, an otherwise healthy patient experiences a sudden pain in the first metatarso-phalangeal joint. The pain may last a few minutes or a few hours. On examination the joint is stiff, tender and painful especially on dorsi flexion. In younger patients there will be no radiological abnormality but as the years pass osteoarthritic changes become increasingly evident. Treatment in the first instance is by applying a metatarsal pad for a week or so. The patient must make sure that his shoes are not too tight and crowding his toes.

Gout

The middle-aged or elderly patient who wakes with a painful tender first metatarso-phalangeal joint almost certainly has gout. These patients are often taking diuretics. While awaiting the results of a serum uric acid estimation, a therapeutic trial of 50 mg indomethacin 3 times a day, will support the diagnosis by bringing rapid relief.

In-growing toe nails

This condition is very common in young men who wear tight socks and shoes and who forget to wash their feet regularly. Incorrect cutting of the toe nails by delving down with the scissors into the grooves at each side of the nail also promotes the complaint. Toe nails should be cut square across the ends. Treatment, if the toe is infected, is usually by removal of the nail under a digital block, and the application of a medicated tulle dressing. Definitive treatment is by wedge re-section of the nail and cauterization of the appropriate section of the nail bed with 80% phenol so that the offending lateral border of the nail does not grow again.

Chapter 18

The treatment of wounds

Introduction

The treatment of wounds is one of the most important parts of the work of an Accident and Emergency Department. The surgeon in charge and the nursing officer must establish a policy and set up a routine which all the staff should follow. The results of this work must be constantly under review so that improvements will come from agreed modifications of the policy. Individual, haphazard variations in the routine usually result in a lowering of the standard of work. The following nine steps form a pattern which should be followed for all wounds. The department should be designed, equipped and staffed so that each step can be taken expeditiously and efficiently.

1. Assessment of the wound.
2. Preparation of the wound area.
3. Anaesthesia.
4. Suturing.
5. Dressing of the wound after suture.
6. Tetanus prevention.
7. Recording of the wound and details of the treatment.
8. Removal of sutures in the Dressing Clinic.
9. Rehabilitation.

The remainder of this chapter is a description of each of these steps in turn, with details of technique where appropriate.

Assessment of the wound

All wounds should be inspected with the patient screened from general view. A friend or relative should only be present if the age or mental state of the patient makes it necessary. Normally, other people do not wish to see bleeding wounds exposed to their gaze. The patient should at least be sitting down. When the wound is severe, involves the lower limb, or is causing undue distress, the patient should be lying down on a couch in a cubicle. The wound may not be large and may pose no threat to life, but it is bound to be a cause of pain and distress to the patient. Kind and gentle consideration will help to alleviate anxiety.

While the nurse removes the First Aid dressing, the doctor can take a brief history. This must elicit the cause, time and circumstance of the accident, and hence the possibility of fractures or injuries to other parts of the body and also of local complications such as the possible presence of foreign bodies, grease or oil or other contaminants. If the injury has been caused by human or animal teeth it carries a risk of serious infection. The patient may be reluctant to admit being in a fight but the presence of a wound of the knuckles of the dominant hand should arouse suspicion.

Patients with major wounds or wounds which require the skill of a specialist surgeon will be admitted to the appropriate ward. Gun-shot wounds and stab wounds of the thorax or abdomen should also be admitted for a full surgical exploration. The management of hand injuries is described in Chapter 13.

The patient should be asked about his previous immunization against tetanus and sensitivity to any antibiotics which may be used.

At this time the doctor should write down the history, a description of the wound–for which a simple sketch is often helpful–and instructions for the patient's management. This will include, if necessary, X-ray for foreign bodies or associated fractures, preliminary preparation of the wound area and the type of anaesthesia to be used during suturing.

Preparation of the wound area

Cleaning of the skin around the wound area will usually be done on the operating table immediately before suture. In some injuries, the surrounding skin may be thickly coated with oil and grease or other dirt, creating a problem for cleaning in the theatre. In these circumstances a proprietory hand cleanser, such as 'Swarfega' is useful. The patient can do the cleaning himself with a sterile, soft nail brush and a sterile bowl containing 1% cetrimide. Since grease may contain anaerobic organisms, especially *Clostridium tetanii,* or, if left in the wound, may produce a painful granuloma, it is particularly important to remove it from the wound. Some crushed fingers are too painful for thorough cleaning until they have been numbed by a local anaesthetic digital nerve block. It is always wise to re-assess the wound after the preliminary cleaning and the necessity for a skin graft may be reconsidered. Hot tar, as used in road works, can be removed either by a proprietory hand cleanser or by olive oil followed by cetrimide toilet. Hot bitumen, as used in roofing, can be left on the skin unless it involves the eyes, mouth or flexion creases. Within 10 days the bitumen will fall off and the skin will usually have healed beneath it. Abrasions with dirt deeply ingrained require scrubbing with cetrimide and a sterile brush under an anaesthetic, otherwise the dirt will produce permanent tattooing. Thorough and painstaking excision of a contaminated or potentially infected wound is mandatory. Only where infection is already established or adequate wound excision is impossible to achieve should antibiotics prove necessary.

Anaesthesia

The majority of wounds sutured in the A & E department can be sutured under local anaesthetic. 1% lignocaine without adrenaline can be infiltrated directly into a clean wound or into the healthy skin around a dirty wound. Children may be helped by oral pre-operative sedation [e.g. 2.5 mg/kg Vallergan, or 2 mg (1–3 year olds) or 4 mg (4–7 year olds) of Valium] and the assistance of a co-operative, stoical parent; but extensive suturing, especially in children who are too young or too afraid to co-operate, requires general anaesthesia. In some wounds of the fingers, a digital nerve block at the base of the finger may be of more use than direct infiltration of local anaesthetic into the wound. In areas of tight tissue tension, where local anaesthetic injection is difficult and painful, mixing an ampoule of hyalase with 10 ml of 1% lignocaine will facilitate the injection, but will of course shorten the duration of the anaesthesia.

Suturing the wound

Suturing a wound must be done as a 'sterile' procedure with the patient comfortably positioned and the area of the wound well illuminated. The operator must then observe the following basic principles:

1. Thoroughly clean the skin around the wound with gauze soaked in 1% cetrimide.

2. Remove all dirt, foreign bodies or dead tissue.
3. Stop any continuing bleeding with a deep stitch or ligature *except* in finger or hand on account of the risk to the nerves that accompany the vessels. Elevate the limb.
4. Bring the remaining tissue into precise apposition using, if necessary, deep absorbable sutures before closing the skin edges in careful alignment.
5. Handle the tissues gently to avoid inflicting further trauma.
6. Tie the sutures firmly to avoid leaving dead space but do not strangle the tissue within the suture–it must have a blood supply in order to heal.
7. Do not suture the wound if undue tension is produced. Rather use either delayed suture, or a skin graft to the defect.
8. When closing the skin, start in the middle of the wound or at jagged corners which will give precise locations on each margin of the wound. This will divide the wound into a number of straight segments which are then halved by each subsequent suture.
9. Remember that skin is living tissue and the wound edges will grow together, provided they have not been inverted, everted or strangled by the sutures.
10. Choice of suture material and size. For deep sutures use catgut. For skin sutures an atraumatic needle should be used of a size appropriate to the wound. Monofilament nylon sutures are recommended for facial wounds because they will be removed after only 3 to 5 days. The same material is indicated for leg wounds, as the sutures should remain *in situ* for 2 weeks. For other wounds, and particularly for children, catgut sutures are preferred because the deep part will dissolve in 10 to 14 days and the exposed part will brush off when the dressing is removed. The suture size varies: for example, 3/0 for a wound on the trunk, leg, an adult upper limb, or scalp; 4/0 for a child's upper limb; 5/0 for an adult face; 6/0 for child's face.

Special wounds

Treatment of wounds of the scalp is described in Chapter 4, wounds of the face and mouth in Chapter 5, and wounds of the hand in Chapter 13.

Deep abrasions and crush injuries

These are caused in two ways. In a road accident the patient slides along the road surface, the superficial skin is abraded and road dirt is embedded in the wound. Under general anaesthesia all dirt must be scrubbed out of the wound with a firm, sterile brush. Loose tags of superficial skin should be cut off. If the dermis is intact, the wound will re-epithelialize with minimal or no scarring. The second type of abrasion is potentially more serious. It occurs when a hand or forearm is trapped between moving rollers in an old wringing machine or in an industrial accident. The skin may still be intact but the shearing force of the rollers, having torn the capillaries beneath the skin, will result in necrosis and sloughing. At the initial examination, if there is no capillary flush in reponse to pressure on the skin, the patient should be referred to a plastic surgeon with a view to excision and skin grafting.

Wounds of the shin

The circulation on the front of the leg is often very poor and wounds are slow to heal. Problems arise most frequently in elderly female patients who lacerate their shin on stairs, the platform of a bus, a coffee table or similar object. The injury often produces a triangular wound with a flap of skin hanging loose at the base. If the length of the flap is more than half the length of its attached base, then necrosis around the edges of the flap is likely. In treating the wound, after thorough cleansing, all loose or damaged fat should be gently cut away. The flap should then be loosely repositioned and the edges gently approximated by applying sterile adhesive strips, covering as much of the wound as is possible without applying any tension. This will often result in the wound remaining incompletely closed. As the oedema subsides and the wound heals this exposed area will diminish in size, and only rarely is a secondary skin graft necessary. Conversely, if at the initial operation the flap is pulled tight by sutures so as to close the whole wound, it probably will slough and a much more extensive grating procedure will be necessary. After the initial operation a non-adhesive, sterile dressing and a firm supporting bandage should be applied. The patient should be advised to reduce his daily activities, but not to stay in bed. When sitting, he should rest the leg on a stool or put it up on a settee or couch. The wound may be re-dressed at weekly intervals.

Dressing of the wound after suture

Dressings are traditional and have a cosmetic value but their real purpose is to protect the wound from further trauma and to rest the part while the wound heals. If the skin is not completely closed, a non-adhesive tulle should be applied to prevent the main dressing sticking to the wound. No dressing should be as tight as to impair the circulation or produce oedema distal to the wound and it is important to ensure that this is so before the patient leaves the department. Adhesive strapping may be used to secure a dressing but care must be taken not to produce a tourniquet effect. A triangular sling may be a useful additional item of dressing to remind the patient to rest an injury of the hand or forearm and to persuade other people to treat him gently for the next few days.

Tetanus prevention

Tetanus still exists and is a constant threat following any open wound. Sportsmen using muddy playing fields and people engaged in gardening or agricultural work, are partiularly at risk.

Active tetanus immunization should be prescribed for all non-immune patients who attend the A & E department for treatment of any wound. It consists of a course of three intramuscular injections of 0.5 ml of adsorbed tetanus toxoid given: one at the first visit, the second after 6 weeks, and the third after 6 months. This gives immunity for 10 years and a booster dose (again 0.5 ml) should be given at or before the expiry of the 10-year period.

When there are indications for giving passive immunization with human tetanus immunoglobulin, a dose of 250 units in 1 ml is given by intramuscular injection. Though extremely rare, an anaphylactic reaction may occur following this injection, and facilities for resuscitation should be available when the injection is given.

In every A & E department there must be a firmly established routine for tetanus prevention. Smith, Laurence and Evans,[*] proposed the following programme which is now widely accepted:

1. All wounds receive surgical toilet (this is the most important single aspect of the treatment programme).
2. Then they divide patients into 4 categories:
   A. Has had a complete course of toxoid or a booster dose within the past 5 years.

[*] Smith, J. W. G., Laurence, D. R. and Evans, D. G. (1975). *Br. Med. J.*, **3,** 453

  B. Has had a complete course of toxoid or a booster dose more than 5 and less than 10 years ago.

  C. Has had a complete course of toxoid or a booster dose more then 10 years ago.

  D. Has not had a complete course of toxoid, or immunity status is unknown.

3. For patients with clean wounds (less than 6 hours old, non-penetrating and negligible tissue damage):

 Category A – nothing more required after surgical treatment of the wound.

 Categories B and C – booster dose of toxoid.

 Category D – complete course of toxoid.

4. For patients with dirty wounds (contaminated, infected, penetrating, more than 6 hours old or with extensive tissue damage):

 Category A – nothing more required after surgical treatment of the wound so far as tetanus protection is concerned.

 Category B – booster dose of toxoid.

 Category C – booster dose of toxoid + human tetanus immunoglobulin.

 Category D – complete course of tetanus toxoid + human tetanus immunoglobulin.

Note: When both toxoid and immunoglobulin are indicated, they can be given at the same time but into different limbs.

Recording of the wound and details of the treatment

The patient's record card will already contain notes on the time, cause and circumstances of the accident. Precise details of the wound or wounds should now be added and again a sketch may be useful to indicate the site and extent of the injuries. The number of sutures and the suture material should be recorded and the presence or absence of other injuries noted. Injections must be recorded, especially tetanus prophylaxis, and the nurse who gives the injection should initial the card. Any prescription given to the patient must also be noted in detail on the record card. It is essential to complete the record card before proceeding to examine or treat another patient.

Removal of sutures in the dressing clinic

Catgut sutures which dissolve or detach in 10–14 days obviate much of the tedious and painful work of removing skin sutures.

This is proving particularly valuable in treating children and patients with hand injuries. However, this does not excuse the surgeon from following up his patients and ensuring that the wounds are well healed. In facial wounds where the sutures will be removed in 3 days, and in leg wounds where the sutures are intended to remain *in situ* for 2 weeks, monofilament nylon sutures are still preferred and these must be removed in the Dressing Clinic.

When patients leave the department after the initial treatment, they should be told to return to any subsequent Dressing Clinic if they are worried; otherwise they should attend after the appropriate number of days according to the site of their injury. Changing the dressing and inspecting the wound before this is meddlesome and should be avoided if possible.

The following figures are given as a guide to the number of days after operation when the wound should be examined and non-absorbable sutures removed if the anticipated degree of healing has occurred:

Face, head and neck	3–5 days
Arm and hand	7 days
Trunk and lower limb	10–14 days

Rehabilitation

After the wound has been inspected and non-absorbable sutures removed, the majority of patients can be discharged from the department and return to their normal activities. However, some patients with moderately severe injuries of the wrist or hand may require a short period of rehabilitation before being able to return to work. In the field of electrotherapy, Diapulse treatment is proving useful in dispersing oedema and thereby reducing pain and stiffness, and this can be given through the dressing from the day of injury. Once the dressing is removed, wax therapy and hand exercises are helpful, and for some patients occupational therapy is indicated to enable them to regain skill and confidence in the use of their hands. Close liaison between the surgeon and the staff of the rehabilitation department will produce excellent results.

Chapter 19

The treatment of burns and scalds

Introduction

A scald is caused by moist heat; a burn may be caused by dry heat, electricity, friction, chemicals or radioactivity. Any of these causes may produce either a 'partial thickness' lesion, where only the epidermis and the superficial part of the dermis is destroyed, or they may produce a 'full thickness' burn in which the lesion extends through the dermis to the subcutaneous tissue. In the partial thickness burn the uninjured, deeper layer of the dermis retains the ability to re-epithelialize the affected area, but in the full thickness burn healing will be by scar tissue unless the affected area is treated surgically by skin grafting. An intermediate condition, a 'deep dermal burn' is described where, although some of the dermis still remains viable, it is so small in quantity that spontaneous healing will be slow and imperfect and for the benefit of the patient skin grafting is indicated.

Clinical distinction between superficial and deep burns is important. The superficial burn is a bright mottled red, painful, tender to touch and blanches on pressure from a sterile gauze. It will form blisters and have a profuse fluid loss. The deep burn is a dusky red or even greyish-white, it is insensitive to touch, does not blanch, and is surprisingly painless. There will be much less free flow of fluid from the surface (*Figure 19.1*).

Patients with extensive burns will have some areas of superficial damage, others with full thickness burns and yet others with the intermediate condition of a deep dermal burn.

Biological effects of skin destruction

The skin is the largest single organ in the body. It performs a number of essential biological functions which are lost when the skin is burned. This causes either immediate or long-term complications which vary in severity depending on the extent and the anatomical site of the burn. These vital functions include:

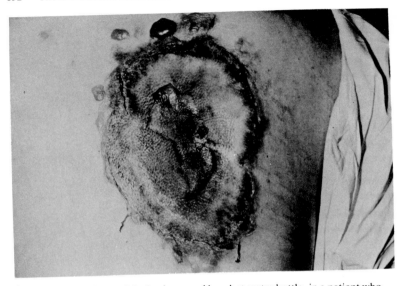

Figure 19.1 Deep burn of the back, caused by a hot-water bottle, in a patient who had taken an overdose

1. *Waterproofing for the body.* As soon as the epidermis is destroyed plasma starts to leak from the burn. If this area is beyond a certain critical percentage of the total body surface, circulatory failure or burns shock will quickly develop unless the lost fluid is replaced by an appropriate infusion.

2. *Bacteria-proofing for the body.* Normally pathogenic bacteria in the atmosphere or on the skin do no harm, but on a fresh burn they will rapidly infect it, delay healing and, if untreated, can produce a systemic toxaemia.

3. *Cutaneous sensation.* The skin is a highly developed sensory organ. In a full-thickness burn this function is permanently destroyed. This is particularly serious when the hands are affected.

4. *Elasticity* to allow for distension and movement. Full thickness burns around the rib cage or over joints can have mechanical disadvantages as the scar tissue will limit movement.

5. *Excretory organ.* The skin normally excretes sweat and sebum and if large areas of the skin are replaced by scar tissue or grafts, then the loss of this excretory function becomes important and body temperature regulation may be impaired.

Assessment of a burned patient

It is essential when a burned patient is brought to the Accident and Emergency Department that the doctor who receives the patients knows immediately what to do. The steps to be followed are:

1. *Check the airway.* Inhalation of flames, hot gases or smoke can result in oedema developing in the upper respiratory passages and tracheotomy may become necessary. The patient will have sufficient physiological problems without the addition of respiratory obstruction and arrangements should be made early for a planned tracheotomy rather than waiting until the patient is obstructed. Soot in the nostrils or burned nasal hairs are warning signs which must never be neglected.
2. *If the patient is in shock,* establish a reliable intravenous line, take a sample of blood for cross-matching, haematocrit, urea and electrolytes, start a plasma drip and introduce a urethral catheter. Then estimate the size of the burn.
3. *If the patient is not in shock,* estimate the percentage of the total skin which is burned. Use Wallace's Rule of Nine (*Figure 19.2*).

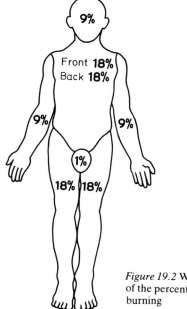

Figure 19.2 Wallace's 'Rule of Nine' for quick assessment of the percentage of the skin which has been injured by burning

Critical limits

In a child or an old person if the percentage burn is 10 per cent or more, or 15 per cent or more in a healthy adult, proceed as in 2 above. If circulatory collapse has not yet occurred it soon will do unless the fluid loss is quickly replaced. These critical limits make intravenous fluid replacement mandatory.

Treatment or prevention of burns shock

This depends on fluid replacement. There are three questions to consider:

1. Which fluids to use.
2. How much to give.
3. How quickly to infuse it.

Unfortunately, there is controversy on all these points but a useful and reliable formula for the first few hours is as follows:

total percentage area of the burn × weight in kilograms ÷ 2 = ml of fluid required in each of 6 periods in the first 36 hours (*Figure 19.3*).

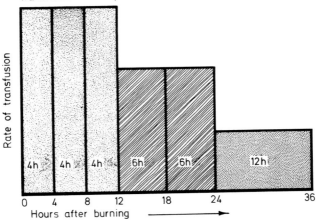

Each rectangle indicates an equal volume of fluid to be transfused in the period shown

Figure 19.3 The 'Mount Vernon' Transfusion Plan. This gives a forward estimate of the patient's colloid requirement. After the first 4 hours, the actual volume of the transfusion will be modified by the patient's response

Example:

A 60 kg patient with a 30 per cent burn will require $(60 \times 30)/2$ = 900 ml of intravenous fluid in each of the 6 periods, making a total transfusion of $6 \times 900 = 5400$ ml within the 36 hours.

It is important to remember that this calculation is to be made from the time of the accident, not from the time when the patient reached hospital. So, if there has been a delay of 2 hours before the patient received treatment, in the above example the patient should receive the first 900 ml within the next 2 hours to put him on schedule.

This formula has proved very satisfactory when the transfusion fluid has been freeze-dried plasma. If Plasma Protein Fraction is used the volume may have to be increased, and if saline or lactated Ringer's solution are used, an even larger increase in the volume is required.

Hourly monitoring of the patient's condition will indicate whether the rate of transfusion requires modification. The following indices are important in this respect:

1. Pulse and blood pressure.
2. Central venous pressure.
3. Jugular vein filling.
4. Pulmonary congestion.
5. Haematocrit.
6. Urine volume and osmolality.

With the widespread catabolic activity which follows an extensive burn a urine output of 0.5–1 ml per minute is necessary to avoid the risk of acute renal failure.

A blood transfusion should form part of the total fluid replacement programme for patients with 10 per cent or more deep burns. A suggested amount is 1 per cent of the patient's normal blood volume for each 1 per cent of deep burn.

Provide analgesia

For large burns intravenous morphine 0.2 mg/kg body weight diluted in 10 ml of saline is given slowly until the pain is relieved. Less extensive burns may need other forms of analgesia, but they usually cease to be painful once they have been hermetically sealed so as to stop evaporation from the burn surface; for example, a sterile occlusive plastic dressing for superficial burns of the trunk or extremities.

Management of the burned patient

If the percentage burn is below the critical levels decide whether the patient can be managed as an out-patient or if he still requires in-patient treatment. Factors favouring in-patient treatment are:

1. Suspected respiratory burns or burns of the face or neck.
2. Burns in the perineal region.
3. Full thickness burns which require skin grafting.
4. Poor general health.
5. Poor home circumstances.

In these or other circumstances which require in-patient care the intitial treatment of the burn must be given in consultation with the surgeon who will be responsible for the patient while in hospital.

If the percentage burn passes the critical limit, under ideal circumstances, the patient should be transferred to a specialized 'Burns Unit' as soon as the airway is assured, a satisfactory drip started and analgesia given.

Local treatment of the burn

Once the necessary steps have been taken to check the airway, replace fluid and relieve pain, local treatment of the burn consists of a gentle cleaning with cetrimide, removing any remnants of burned clothing and cutting off any strands of dead epithelium which are hanging loose. Small intact blisters may be cleaned and left; large ones, which are likely to burst should be opened with sterile scissors. If the burn is full thickness and passes right round the whole circumference of the trunk, limb or digit, it should be incised longitudinally to prevent occlusion of the circulation or respiratory embarrassment as oedema forms within the burn.

For extensive burns on one aspect only of the trunk or a limb, the 'open-method' of treatment is probably the best. The patient is nursed on a freshly laundered sheet with the burn exposed to light and a current of warm air. The plasma exuding from the burn will soon coagulate and the coagulum then forms a barrier against further fluid loss and also against infection.

For those parts of the body such as the inner aspects of the arm or legs, where rubbing will break down the coagulum, we have found the application of a sterile sheet of adhesive plastic film to be very useful. This application has a further value in that patients can wash over it. As the burn heals beneath it, the film will gradually become detached. For children with burns of the trunk, this method is particularly useful as it avoids using bulky bandages which tend to slip out of place, become soiled and restrict the child's movements.

For small full thickness burns which do not require excision and grafting, and for neglected burns, Flamazine is a useful local application. It is spread liberally over the burn, covered with a tulle dressing and gauze, and secured with bandages.

Once the burn has been effectively dressed it is meddlesome to keep taking the dressing off. The patient should be seen again within 2 days to ensure that he is comfortable and that the dressing is still dry. The next visits are on the fifth and tenth days for the dressing to be changed, preferably at a separate clinic. By then superficial burns should be healed and any necessary further treatment can be considered for deep burns.

Use of antibiotics and tetanus immunization

An extensive study of burns managed on an out-patient basis has shown that only 3 per cent become infected. These few cases can be treated by cetrimide toilet followed by the application of a medicated tulle. The use of systemic antibiotics is only indicated in burns extensive enough to require resuscitation.

Patients with deep burns should be immunized against tetanus (*see* Chapter 18).

Prevention of joint contracture

Full thickness or deep dermal burns in the region of joints will, if left to heal naturally, form scar tissue which will then contract and limit the range of movement of the joint. Splinting the joints will diminish this tendency. This is particularly important in the hands which should be supported with the metacarpo-phalangeal joint flexed and the interphalangeal joints extended. This position prevents contracture of the collateral ligaments of these joints.

Skin grafting

Patients with full thickness burns or deep dermal burns, especially if near a joint, should have the benefit of a plastic surgeon's opinion. Recent trends have been towards applying skin grafts much sooner after the accident. It is preferable for the plastic surgeon to see a patient and decide that grafting will not be necessary than for him to be presented for the first time with a patient with established joint contractures for whom surgery will have to be much more extensive because of delay in seeking surgical replacement of the burned skin.

Burns from various causes

Electricity burns

The burn may be only part of the problem of electrocution. Clearly, if cardiac arrest has occurred, cardiopulmonary resuscitation takes precedence. The distinctive feature of these burns is that the surface area of the burn may be relatively small but there is often a track of dead tissue along the line of passage of the current. This burn in depth, rather than in area, creates surgical problems which will often necessitate admission to hospital and may require surgical treatment for what, on the surface, appears to be a small injury.

Friction burns

These are of two distinct varieties. Firstly, where the patient slides across an abrading surface, as for instance following a motor cycle accident, road dirt will be embedded in the burns and must be scrubbed out under general anaesthetic. Secondly, where some part of the patient is trapped between moving rollers. Here the skin will be abraded and scuffed but more important the dermis may have been sheared off the subcutaneous tissue and so have lost its blood supply. Such a friction burn may not look too serious when first seen but subsequently there can be extensive skin necrosis and a plastic surgeon's opinion should be obtained early in the management of these patients.

Chemical burns

The medical staff and nursing staff working in an A & E Department should be kept informed of any special risks from chemical industries in their locality or of chemical products being regularly transported through their area. Most chemical burns arise in accidents in the home or in school laboratories and can be treated by copious washing with tap water. Corneal burns, after thorough irrigation, should be treated with mydriatic drops and local antibiotics and be referred for an ophthalmic opinion (*see* Chapter 6).

Radioactivity burns

In Britain comprehensive arrangements for the reception and treatment of patients involved in incidents involving radioactivity are described in the *Health Circular HC(76)52* issued in November 1976, and all Accident Departments should have a copy available for immediate reference.

When the patient is too ill to be taken to one of the specially designated hospitals he will be taken to the nearest A & E Department, and the following advice from the circular should be followed. 'If time is available, the following preparations should be made before the patient arrives at the hospital:

1. An area, not necessarily within the casualty department, should be set aside (the 'dirty' area) for the reception of casualties and, if the floor is not easily cleaned, it should be covered with plastic sheeting or heavy duty paper. Newspaper can be used if nothing else is available.
2. Protective clothing should be issued for all staff who will handle the patient.
3. A plentiful supply of paper towels and tissue should be available.
4. Large polythene or paper bags will be needed for the collection of the patient's clothing and contaminated equipment etc.
5. An area should be cleared where the ambulance can wait for monitoring and possible decontamination.
6. A limited number of staff should be appointed to handle the patient and a person should be designated to log the movements of any of those staff who must leave the 'dirty' area after the casualties have arrived, in order to minimize the difficulty of tracing contamination.
7. If other areas of the hospital become involved in handling the patient, e.g. a theatre or Intensive Care Unit, similar arrangements should be made for these areas as appropriate.
8. A person should be designated to deal with enquiries, public relations, etc.

The following initial decontamination procedures should be followed:

1. Experience has shown that washing with soap and water will effectively remove contaminated material from the skin in most cases. Initial treatment and any necessary washing to remove as much of the suspected contamination as practicable should be done in the 'dirty' area.

2. Open wounds should be irrigated. Special care needs to be taken in the cleaning of areas near the eye and in preventing the spread of possible contamination to other parts of the body.

3. It will usually be possible to seek further expert advice from a designated hospital before proceeding beyond the initial treatment stage, and it is inadvisable to excise wounds, unless contamination is obvious or unless surgically indicated, before monitoring assistance is available.'

Chapter 20

The treatment of the acute abscess

Basic pathology of abscess formation and response to treatment

An abscess is a collection of pus surrounded by a 'pyogenic membrane'. As the abscess grows in size the inner surface of the membrane sloughs and liquifies to add to the volume of pus, and the outer surface enlarges as the body continues the battle to localize and contain the area of infection. The membrane has two important properties: it prevents the spread of toxic products or live bacteria from the abscess into the general circulation and it allows leucocytes to pass from the circulation into the abscess to ingest the bacteria. Unfortunately, from the point of view of therapy, antibiotics carried in the blood stream do not traverse the pyogenic membrane and so cannot play any direct role in the treatment of an abscess unless this barrier is first breached by surgical intervention.

Before the advent of antibiotics it was common surgical practice to delay incision of an abscess until it was bulging under the skin. To hasten this process, poultices or fomentations were used to 'draw' the abscess to the surface. Then, once it was 'ripe' or 'pointing', it was realized from empirical observation that incision would allow the pus to drain away without infecting the surrounding tissues. At the beginning of the antibiotic era Maurice Ellis showed that if an intramuscular injection of an effective antibiotic was one-half to one hour before incision, the risk of spreading the infection to surrounding tissues by operating early in the evolution of the abscess, was completely eradicated. Consequently, poultices and fomentations were no longer needed and they now have no role to play in the modern treatment of an acute abscess. If pus is judged to be present, arrangements should be made immediately to evacuate it under an antibiotic cover.

Ellis continued this pioneer work by showing that, after incision, curettage of the wall of the abscess resulted in antibiotic-laden blood filling the cavity. Then, if any loculi were broken down and all pus and debris removed, the area became sterile under the influence of the antibiotic and so was amenable to primary closure. Prior to this advance in surgical technique a surgeon, having evacuated the pus from an abscess cavity, felt obliged to pack the cavity with a 'wick' or ribbon gauze to prevent the cavity closing at the surface before the deeper portion had healed. The essential point in the Ellis technique is that the cavity should be occluded by deep sutures passing right round it to obliterate any dead space. Healing then takes place simultaneously throughout the whole area by first intention, as in a laceration.

A further advantage of this technique is that, as all the cellular and humeral elements necessary for wound healing are already on site in abundance, there is no lag phase in the speed of wound healing. Whereas a clean surgical incision may require 8 days before the sutures can be safely removed, an incision in a formerly infected, but now sterile area, will heal in 5 days. Provided the surgery is correctly performed and the antibiotic is effective against the causal organism, the treatment can be used on an out-patient basis. Under optimum conditions the patient only makes two visits to hospital, one for the initial surgery, and the second to have the sutures removed after 5 days. Healing will be delayed in those patients who waited until the abscess was 'pointing' before coming for treatment. The same technique is applicable but there will be some superficial skin necrosis, the skin having been damaged by the inflammatory process. If pointing has proceeded to actual bursting through the skin, a small abscess will then heal spontaneously but a large one still justifies a full surgical curettage and suture under antibiotic cover, otherwise a sinus may result. Failure of this technique to produce rapid and complete healing usually means that one or more of the following errors has been committed:

1. The antibiotic has inadvertently been forgotten.
2. All loculi were not broken down.
3. Slough, dead tissue or pyogenic membrane were left in the cavity.
4. The sutures did not adequately obliterate the cavity.
5. The organisms were insensitive to the antibiotic.

Special sites of abscess formation

Infection in the hand

Delay in operating on abscesses in the infected hand is still far too common. Very early infection of the hand before a definite abscess is formed may respond to antibiotic treatment. However, if the patient's sleep has been disturbed the previous night by a throbbing pain, pus is almost certainly present and incision under an antibiotic cover should be planned immediately. Physical examination will show the classical signs of local heat, redness, pain and swelling, and occasionally the added complications of lymphangitis and axillary lymphadenitis. If the patient gives a history of frequent soft tissue infection, his general health should be investigated. Diabetes, leukaemia or an underlying focus of infection such as osteomyelitis must be considered. Asian immigrants in Britain sometimes present with a rapidly evolving tuberculous infection of the soft tissues which fortunately responds quickly to appropriate antibiotic treatment once the correct diagnosis is made.

Anaesthesia

For infections in the distal half of a finger a digital nerve block is indicated: 2 ml of 1% lignocaine, without adrenaline, are injected into the region of the digital nerves at the base of the finger. These nerves run on each side of the finger midway between palmar and dorsal aspects. After injection it may take up to 15 minutes for the anaesthetic to penetrate to the centre of the nerve and so anaesthetize the sensory fibres which arise at the finger tip. For more proximally situated infections in the hand, general or regional anaesthesia is necessary.

Paronychia

This very common condition, an infection at the side of the nail, commonly called a 'whitlow' may arise from three separate causes: usually bacterial, occasionally fungal and very occasionally viral.

Acute paronychia. This is usually due to a staphylococcal infection. To effect a cure, under a digital block, an incision is made parallel to the edge of the nail and 1 mm away from it. A swab is taken from the pus, pyogenic membrane and any dead tissue are curetted away and then the wound edges will fall into place. A firm dressing will obliterate any dead space. The condition is usually fully healed in 4 days.

Sub-acute paronychia. This condition has usually been present for 2–3 weeks before the patient seeks treatment and it is not as painful as acute paronychia. It usually affects several fingers at the same time. The cause is a fungus infection which will respond to applications of an anti-fungal ointment and an occlusive dressing.

'Herpetic whitlow'

This is an occupational hazard of nurses, especially those nursing tracheostomy patients. Nurses doing tracheal toilet or dressings should wear disposable gloves. The lesion starts as a vesicle surrounded by inflammation. In succeeding days further vesicles appear and the condition becomes increasingly painful. Incision will fail to demonstrate any pus but may result in secondary bacterial infection. Antibiotics have no effect on the virus and the treatment is to dress the finger with 5% idoxuridine or 5% acyclodir daily for 3–4 days.

Pulp space infections

These are extremely painful. The soft tissues and skin which form the pulp at the ends of the fingers have a very rich sensory innervation; consequently, patients tend to come early for treatment. A surgical approach should be made from under the cover of the hood of the projecting finger nail. In this way scarring across the sensitive skin of the pulp is avoided. All dead tissue must be carefully removed because any lingering infection may result in infection spreading to the bones of the terminal phalanx and producing an osteomyelitis. After adequate surgery, suturing is rarely necessary; a firm dressing will hold the tissues in place and occlude any dead space. Healing should be complete within a week.

Subcutaneous abscess

These abscesses can occur anywhere on the fingers or hand and the acute paronychia and pulp space infections are no more than a subcutaneous abscess in a particularly common site. The principles of treatment are the same. Incision should be made in the line of the skin creases and care must be taken to evacuate all the pus. Occasionally a 'collar stud' abscess may develop with superficial and deep pockets of pus connected only by a narrow sinus. If only the superficial pus is evacuated the condition will fail to respond to the treatment.

Web space infection

This infection occurs at the base of the finger on the palmar aspect. The infection spreads quickly into the webs of the finger, proximally into the palm for about 2 cm, and distally into the proximal segment of the finger. Redness and oedema usually develop early on the dorsum of the hand. Indeed, the patient often shows the red swollen dorsum of the hand as the main area of complaint, but questioning and physical examination will establish that the centre of infection is on the palmar aspect at the base of the finger. Under general anaesthesia an incision is made in the proximal palmar crease of the finger, care being taken not to incise too deeply and involve the flexor tendon sheath. After expressing the pus and gently curetting the lining of the abscess, a firm dressing is applied. The natural semiflexed position of the fingers apposes the skin edges and collapses the cavity. Healing will be complete in 4–5 days, whereas if an incision is made in the finger web, even if it is sutured, it would take well over a week to heal.

Suppurative tenosynovitis

This condition is important and demands urgent treatment. The original wound is often trivial and may have passed unnoticed. In the early stages pus develops in the fibrous flexor sheath of a finger. Gradually the tension in the sheath equals or exceeds the pressure in the surrounding arterioles and capillaries and the blood supply to the tendons is occluded. If the sheath is not promptly decompressed, the tendons may undergo necrosis and the patient is then left with a useless stiff finger. The usual presentation is of a painful throbbing, tender, sausage-shaped swelling on the volar aspect of the finger extending into the distal half of the palm. The finger is held semiflexed, extension of the finger is painful and further flexion is limited by the swelling. Treatment is by operation under general anaesthesia and a tourniquet. After a pre-operative intramuscular injection of an effective antibiotic, one incision is made in the mid-palmar crease and a second one in the flexor crease of the distal interphalangeal joint. This allows the flexor sheath to be opened both proximally and distally. A No. 4 FG plastic catheter is now passed along the sheath to decompress it and to irrigate it with an antibiotic solution. Once a free flow of the antibiotic solution has been established the catheter can be withdrawn and the incisions closed. Antibiotic therapy should be continued orally for 4–5 days while the nature of the infecting organism and its sensitivity is established. Later the patient may benefit from wax baths and exercises in the Physiotherapy Department to help regain the full use of the finger.

Palmar space infections

Infections localized to the thenar, mid-palmar or hypothenar spaces are now very rarely seen. They probably only arise as a complication of a neglected or inadequately treated infection elsewhere in the hand. The principles of treatment are the same: incision and curettage under an antibiotic cover.

Carbuncle

This type of infection occurs on the dorsum of the hand and fingers in association with hair follicles. Antibiotics will not heal the condition but may prevent the infection spreading to other adjacent hair follicles. A hygroscopic dressing such as magnesium sulphate paste will help to draw the pus and slough out of the follicles. If resolution is slow surgical removal of the slough is indicated.

Infected sebaceous cyst

This is a common condition in any hair bearing area. Treatment by antibiotics and aspiration may be attempted but often incision, curettage and suture is required.

Axillary abscesses

These are very common especially in patients who shave the axilla and use a strong deodorant. The Ellis treatment of incision, curettage and primary sutures under an antibiotic cover is eminently suitable and, provided it is properly executed, there is no place for the use of packs or wicks which, being in themselves foreign bodies, can only serve to delay healing.

Breast abscesses

The incidence of this abscess has declined greatly in the last decade, probably because of improved methods of suppressing lactation in the post-partum period. Because of the amenable anatomical structure of the breast, the Ellis treatment probably benefits these patients more than any others. A large breast abscess may contain 50–100 ml of pus and an enthusiastic but ill-informed surgeon can pack the cavity with several metres of ribbon gauze. Packing a breast abscess in this way can perpetuate it for weeks. Using the Ellis technique, with an incision radiating away from the nipple followed by a comprehensive curettage, the abscess will heal in 5 days especially because the breast is so amenable to the use of deep obliterative sutures. There can be no doubt that this method should be used in all acute breast abscesses.

Occasionally a rapidly growing, anaplastic carcinoma of breast may look line an abscess. If, on incision, no pus is found but rather tumour-like tissue and necrotic fluid, a biopsy should be taken and further surgical advice obtained.

Ano-rectal abscesses

This common condition has provided the most testing challenge to the Ellis* technique of abscess treatment and it is this type of abscess which has been most thoroughly investigated in assessing the value of the method. The patient is usually middle-aged (30–50 years) and comes to the Accident and Emergency Department complaining of a throbbing, painful swelling around the anus which has kept him awake for the past 2 or 3 nights. The physical signs depend on the degree of evolution of the abscess. In the early stages, there may be nothing more than an area of tender induration but, if sleep has been disturbed, pus is present and surgery should be arranged immediately.

The traditional method of treatment for this abscess is to make an incision radiating away from the anal orifice to release the pus, then to de-roof the cavity by making a second incision at right angles to the first one. The edges of the skin are trimmed with scissors and haemostasis achieved using diathermy coagulation; the cavity is then packed with ribbon gauze soaked in an antiseptic solution. Post-operatively the patient remains in hospital and the pack is changed daily until healing is sufficiently advanced in 5 or 6 days' time for subsequent dressings to be done by the District Nurse or by the patient himself at home.

Using the Ellis method, the patients are treated on an out-patient basis but the surgical procedure requires at least as much care and operative skill as does the traditional method. Half to one hour before surgery, the patient is given an intramuscular injection of an antibiotic. The choice of antibiotic is important: it must be effective against anaerobic organisms such as *Bacteroides* as well as the staphylococcus because a variety of organisms can be responsible for the infection. Then, under a general anaesthetic the patient is placed in the lithotomy position, the perineum is shaved, a radial incision is made and a bacteriological swab is taken of the first pus to flow out. The gloved index finger is inserted to determine whether the abscess is 'perianal' with an intact ischio-rectal fascia above it, or 'ischio-rectal' with a

*Ellis, M. (1960). Incision and primary suture of abscesses of the anal region. *Proc. R. Soc. Med., **53**, 652

perforation of the fascia. In the latter instance, this perforation must be enlarged to allow complete evacuation of the pus and pyogenic membrane lying above the fascia. After thorough curettage all remaining debris is removed by a gauze toilet of the cavity. Then, using a 2/0 monofilament nylon suture on a large half circle needle, the left index finger is placed in the cavity to gauge the depth to which the sutures must be passed to occlude the cavity; two or three sutures are introduced before any are tied. Finally, a sterile dressing is applied and after recovering from the anaesthetic the patient can return home. If the dressing becomes soiled it can be changed at home or at the hospital. On the fifth or sixth day the wound is inspected. Usually by this time, because all the swelling has subsided, the sutures are lying loose and can easily be removed. The patient should now be instructed to bath daily and to change the dressing himself if there is any further drainage. The patient may now be discharged or may require one further out-patient visit.

We have previously published a retrospective two-year follow-up of 100 patients treated in this way. This shows a 78 per cent success rate without any recurrence of symptoms, 15 per cent of patients had another abscess form within the succeeding 2 years and 7 per cent developed an anal fistula. More recently we have co-operated with Leaper *et al.** in a prospective study of 219 patients treated on a randomized basis either by the traditional method or by the Ellis method. *Table 20.1* indicates the advantages for the patient of the Ellis method.

TABLE 20.1. Comparison of the results of a randomized trial of the treatment of ano-rectal abscess (*see* text)

	Traditional method	Ellis method
Number of patients	109	110
Average no. of days as an in-patient	4	0
Average no. of days off work	31	8
Average no. of days to full healing	35	10

*Leaper, D. J., Page, R. E., Rosenberg, I. L., Wilson, D. H. and Goligher, J. C. (1976). A controlled study comparing treatment of idiopathic ano-rectal abscess with that of incision, curettage and primary suture under systemic antibiotic cover. *Dis. Colon Rectum*, **19,** 46

Further reading

BLICK, P. W. H., FLOWERS, M. W., MARSDEN, A. K., WILSON, D. H., GHONEIM, A. T. M. (1980). Antibiotics in surgical treatment of acute abscesses. *Br. med. J.*, **281**, 111–112

JONES, N. A. G. and WILSON, D. H. (1976) The treatment of acute abscesses by incision, curettage and primary suture under antibiotic cover. *Br. J. Surg.*, **63**, 499–501

WILSON, D. H. (1964). The late results of ano-rectal abscess treated by incision, curettage and primary suture under antibiotic cover. *Br. J. Surg.*, **51**, 828

A 16 mm cine film of the surgical technique is available from Leeds University Television Unit, Leeds 2.

Chapter 21

The acute abdomen

The diagnosis of acute surgical disease in the abdomen forms one of the most fascinating parts of the work of the Emergency Department. Abdominal pain may be accompanied by other symptoms such as fever, nausea or vomiting, diarrhoea or frequency of micturition, but it is usually the pain which is the presenting symptom. A careful history and examination, and certain basic investigations are required to diagnose or exclude an acute surgical cause for the pain. With years of experience a senior doctor will improve his diagnostic acumen, learning which questions to ask and how much significance to attach to the answers. A junior doctor, especially if working under pressure or through the night hours, is more likely to make a wrong decision which could have disastrous consequences for the patient.

A study of the diagnostic accuracy of junior doctors working unaided showed that their provisional diagnosis was correct for only 42 per cent of patients admitted to hospital with an 'acute abdomen'. The introduction of an 'Acute Abdominal Chart' or diagnostic check-list (*Figure 21.1*) enabled them to develop a systematized method of history-taking and physical examination and to avoid forgetting to ask certain essential questions. The immediate results of this innovation were to raise the diagnostic accuracy from 42 per cent to 61 per cent and also to increase significantly the doctor's ability to send a patient home with a confident and correct decision that their symptoms did not require hospital treatment.

In Leeds it has been shown that it is practical to use a computer to store the diagnostic information gained from many hundreds of patients with acute abdominal disease. Then the details of the signs and symptoms from a new patient can be compared with this data base and the computer will make a diagnostic prediction which is at least as reliable as that of the most experienced clinician. We are not suggesting that the computer can replace the clinician, but we do consider that it can be of great help in improving the level of diagnostic accuracy to 70 per cent or higher.

Abdominal Pain Chart

NAME		REG NUMBER	
MALE FEMALE AGE		FORM FILLED BY	
PRESENTATION (999, GP, etc)		DATE	TIME

PAIN

SITE

ONSET

PRESENT

RADIATION

AGGRAVATING FACTORS
movement
coughing
respiration
food
other
none

RELIEVING FACTORS
lying still
vomiting
antacids
food
other
none

PROGRESS
better
same
worse
DURATION

TYPE
intermittent
steady
colicky

SEVERITY
moderate
severe

HISTORY

NAUSEA
   yes   no

VOMITING
   yes   no

ANOREXIA
   yes   no

PREV INDIGESTION
   yes   no

JAUNDICE
   yes   no

BOWELS
normal
constipation
diarrhoea
blood
mucus

MICTURITION
normal
frequency
dysuria
dark
haematuria

PREV SIMILAR PAIN
   yes   no

PREV ABDO SURGERY
   yes   no

DRUGS FOR ABDO PAIN
   yes   no

♀ LMP

pregnant

Vag. discharge

dizzy/faint

EXAMINATION

MOOD
normal
distressed
anxious

SHOCKED
   yes   no

COLOUR
normal
pale
flushed
jaundiced
cyanosed

TEMP   PULSE

BP

ABDO MOVEMENT
normal
poor/nil
peristalsis

SCAR
   yes   no

DISTENSION
   yes   no

TENDERNESS

REBOUND
   yes   no

GUARDING
   yes   no

RIGIDITY
   yes   no

MASS
   yes   no

MURPHY'S
   +ve   −ve

BOWEL SOUNDS
normal   absent   + + +

RECTAL — VAGINAL TENDERNESS
left
right
general
mass
none

INITIAL DIAGNOSIS & PLAN

RESULTS
amylase
blood count (WBC)
computer
urine
X-ray
other

DIAG & PLAN AFTER INVEST

(time   )

DISCHARGE DIAGNOSIS

History and examination of other systems on separate case notes

UPS 4462 7 82

Figure 21.1 Diagnostic check-list designed for computer analysis of the signs and symptoms of acute abdominal pain

In ideal circumstances, quite apart from these methods, a junior doctor should be present in the theatre when a patient's abdomen is explored so that he can see for himself the significance of the signs and symptoms he has elicited.

Acute appendicitis

In temperate climates, the commonest acute surgical lesion producing abdominal pain is acute appendicitis. The population at large, particularly anxious mothers and school teachers, nearly always think of appendicitis as the cause of abdominal pain, especially if the pain is on the right side. Acute appendicitis is predominantly a young person's disease and when it occurs in a small child or an old person, it is more difficult to diagnose. Intussusception in the child and malignancy in the elderly are possible alternative diagnoses.

Signs and symptoms

There are seven cardinal features of acute appendicitis:

1. The pain was originally in the centre of the abdomen but later it moved to the right lower quadrant.
2. The pain is made worse by coughing or by sitting up unaided from a lying position.
3. Anorexia, nausea and vomiting–usually all three are present.
4. The patient is flushed even though the temperature is only slightly raised (37–38 °C).
5. There is tenderness on palpation localized to the right lower quadrant.
6. Rebound tenderness and guarding are present in the right lower quadrant.
7. Rectal examination elicits pain on the right side.

Unless at least two of these features are present the patient is very unlikely to have appendicitis and can probably be sent home. If two features are present appendicitis is possible and the patient should be kept under observation. The presence of three or more features makes the diagnosis almost certain.

Differential diagnoses

More than half of all the patients who come to an Emergency Department complaining of acute abdominal pain will be found to have 'non-specific abdominal pain'. They do not require surgery and most of them can be safely returned home. However, if the patient is over 50 years of age there is a 10 per cent possibility that their pain is due to a malignancy. Further features suggesting an undiagnosed cancer are that they have had a previous, less severe, bout of pain; this time the pain has been present for 2–3 days but has been intermittent. A recent change in bowel habit and any loss in weight further support the necessity of referral for investigation of a possible gastrointestinal neoplasm.

While remembering that common things occur commonly and that a case of acute appendicitis should never be missed, there are other diagnoses which may be confused with appendicitis. Lower lobe pneumonia or pleurisy on the right side of the chest may simulate the pain of appendicitis, but physical examination and a chest X-ray should clearly distinguish between the two. Myocardial infarction is an increasingly common cause of acute pain and its occurrence is increasing in young middle-aged people. Even though the description of the pain may be vague and the radiation bizarre a careful history and physical examination should avoid any confusion with appendicitis. Perforated peptic ulcer, acute cholecystitis and intestinal obstruction are discussed later in this chapter.

The diarrhoea and vomiting of gastroenteritis may produce severe spasms of abdominal pain with an intermittent dull ache and generalized tenderness over the abdomen. In children a pelvic appendicitis may produce diarrhoea, but the rectal examination should establish this diagnosis. An inflamed appendix lying close to the urinary tract may, by inflammatory irritation, produce frequency and dysuria. Tenderness in the loin or a tender palpable kidney with heavily infected urine will suggest pyelitis rather than appendicitis as the cause of these urinary symptoms.

Negro children with sickle cell disease may suffer from acute abdominal pain due to small mesenteric infarcts, and older people with arteriosclerosis may have larger infarcts producing intestinal obstruction.

Drug addicts may simulate the pain of acute appendicitis or other abdominal disease. Their insistent demands for an analgesic injection should raise one's suspicion. If there is a previous operation scar a gesture at ringing the previous hospital for further information often precipitates their prompt departure.

Intestinal obstruction

The majority of patients with intestinal obstruction present themselves to the doctor because of pain. There is a smaller group of patients for whom vomiting is the principal complaint.

Clinical features

A history of intermittent, colicky abdominal pain should raise the possibility of intestinal obstruction and other symptoms must be sought to confirm or refute this diagnosis.

If vomiting is present as well as recurring colicky pain, it is certainly confirmatory evidence, but the absence of vomiting or only trivial vomiting does not rule out obstruction. Vomiting may be quite late in appearance with obstruction at the lower end of the large bowel, but can be a very early symptom in proximal small bowel obstruction.

If present, constipation is confirmatory evidence, but its absence does not rule out obstruction especially when the site of the lesion is in the small bowel. It is always necessary to enquire about it or a patient with colicky pain and vomiting may omit to mention that he has diarrhoea and thus a case of gastroenteritis may be mis-diagnosed as obstruction, especially as in the severe case fluid levels may be seen on X-ray.

The patient may volunteer that there is a painful swelling, suggesting a strangulated hernia as the cause of the obstruction, but the absence of a painful lump does not rule out the diagnosis of obstruction. Intestinal adhesions, mesenteric infarction, volvulus, an internal hernia, tumour or, in the elderly, diverticulitis or chronic constipation may be the cause.

Physical examination

The suspicion of intestinal obstruction having been raised by the history, the abdomen is examined with the patient lying flat with a pillow under the head, and the hips and knees slightly flexed. The whole of the abdomen must be uncovered or the presence of a lump around the groins may be missed. A small femoral hernia in a corpulent female is easily overlooked. A quick inspection of the groins may show an obvious lump, but at this stage palpation should wait. Inspection is an important part of the examination. With obstruction, the abdomen is always distended to a greater or lesser degree and, excluding a strangulated hernia with a painful, tender external lump, obstruction cannot really be diagnosed without distension. But the distension of obstruction is caused by gas in coils of gut, and since all coils are not equally distended with gas, the distension of the abdomen will be asymmetrical. With a history of intermittent colicky pain with vomiting or constipation, as soon as the abdomen is uncovered look for irregular distension. If it is present, sit down and watch it. After a while the irregular pattern will alter: small mounds of distension will appear which were not there a minute before, while other distended mounds will disappear. The period of observation need not be longer than 5 minutes at the outside to be sure that these changes in distension are taking place.

Further physical examination is aimed at finding out the cause of the obstruction. After palpation of the groins, loins and abdomen, rectal examination is a mandatory part of the examination. In old people this can reveal a mass of impacted faeces; manual evacuation, if necessary under anaesthetic, is followed by a dramatic recovery. In other patients rectal examination may reveal a tumour as the cause of the obstruction, or the rectum may be dilated and empty, which is confirmatory evidence of the diagnosis already made.

Radiological examination

This should follow the completion of the physical examination and is never a substitute for it. Two views are taken: one with the patient supine and one in the erect position. The appearance of fluid levels on the erect film, except for a patient with severe gastroenteritis or a child under 2 years of age, are confirmatory evidence of intestinal obstruction. Valvulae conniventes seen to traverse the full diameter of the small bowel or the appearance of haustrations on the large bowel are further confirmatory radiological signs.

All patients with intestinal obstruction require urgent admission to hospital and they usually require a laparotomy.

Intussusception

These cases are often very difficult to diagnose. The typical case occurs in an infant around the age of 1 year. Boys are affected more often than girls. The baby cannot complain of pain, but the mother seeks help because, from out of the blue, the infant has an attack of screaming as if it were in pain. There may be vomiting and there may be the classical redcurrant jelly motions. Vomiting is so frequent with any sick infant that no special diagnostic weight can be attached to it. The 'redcurrant jelly' passed per rectum makes the diagnosis of intussusception very probable, but some forms of gastroenteritis can produce this, as can bacillary dysentery.

Usually with intussusception, the child looks quite well between the attacks of screaming. By contrast, the child with gastroenteritis or dysentery looks toxic, especially if the symptoms have persisted for 24 hours or more. Attempting to examine the abdomen of a restless crying baby will probably not reveal any valuable information. The examiner must use all his wits to see that the child is lying relaxed and quiet. It usually pays to tell the mother exactly what is required. Playing with the child, nursing it or talking to it may not succeed. The doctor should leave the room and come back quietly when the child is relaxed and then place a warm gentle hand on the abdomen to feel for the typical sausage-shaped lump. The lump is usually palpable in the epigastrium and may be felt as soon as the hand is placed there. If it is not felt immediately, the hand should stay there and wait. After a short time, if there is an intussusception, a wave of peristalsis will make the gut contract and the tumour will be felt. Only too often just as the peristalsis comes on the child feels pain, starts to cry, the abdominal wall contracts and the chance of feeling the tumour goes. The examination may have to be repeated several times, but if there is an intussusception, a tumour can usually be felt eventually and the diagnosis established.

Only when the abdominal examination is complete should a rectal examination be performed. If there has already been a redcurrant jelly motion, it is not really necessary. Sometimes some of this characteristic stool is seen on the tip of the examining finger. Occasionally the apex of the intussusception may be palpated in the rectum.

A skilled radiologist will be able to help when the diagnosis is in doubt by giving a barium enema and occasionally, in an early case, the enema can be used as a means of therapy to reduce the intussusception.

Perforated peptic ulcer

The diagnosis of the typical perforated peptic ulcer is one of the easiest to make of all the acute abdominal catastrophes. A history of severe abdominal pain of recent onset, combined with generalized abdominal tenderness and board-like rigidity of the abdominal muscles, makes an unmistakable clinical picture. The patient lies immobile and the typical steely grey facies, once recognized, suggests the diagnosis as the doctor approaches the bedside. As these perforations can occur at any time, the severity of the pain may cause the patient to come to hospital from home, the street or from work without waiting to be seen by the general practitioner.

The more difficult case is the patient who is known to have a duodenal ulcer of long standing and who comes to hospital with a severe exacerbation of pain often after imbibing a quantity of alcohol. In some of these patients, the ulcer has perforated and the typical picture described above is present. In others there has only been a small localized leak of duodenal contents which is then sealed off by the omentum and surrounding viscera. Radiological examination may be particularly helpful in determining the diagnosis for these patients. The film of the abdomen taken in the erect position will show air under the diaphragm in some 70 per cent of patients. As little as 20 ml of free air in the peritoneal cavity will produce the characteristic crescent-shaped gas shadow between diaphragm and liver. In the remainder of these patients the intake of alcohol has produced an acute gastritis, but there has been no perforation. The pain may be so severe as to be confused with a myocardial infarction. If there has been a leak of duodenal contents this may irritate the left leaf of the diaphragm and produce pain behind the left shoulder which can further confuse the diagnosis. An ECG should be performed but its interpretation may be equivocal. Physical examination, repeated every 30 minutes, will soon establish the true diagnosis.

Haematemesis and melaena

The clinical symptoms of acute gastrointestinal bleeding are that a patient begins to feel unwell, becomes nauseated, starts to sweat and looks pale. Then, after a variable period of time from minutes to a few hours, the patient vomits up either fresh blood or coffee ground material. Subsequently he may pass a large, soft, tarry, melaena stool. In the Emergency Department resuscitation takes precedence over any effort to determine the site of the bleeding. An intravenous line must be established. Even if the patient is not shocked at this stage he may become so. The fluid infused will be determined by the general condition of the patient. Saline may suffice in the mild case while cross-matched blood is awaited. Occasionally, in the most severe cases, Group O negative blood may have to be used until cross-matched blood becomes available. In recent years the improvement in skills and equipment for fibre optic gastroenteroscopy has considerably improved the prognosis in the management of these patients.

Acute cholecystitis

Traditionally it is taught that patients with cholecystitis are fair, fat, forty and female. Some may be, but our studies show that, although the condition is unusual under 40 years of age, its incidence increases with age from the middle years of life onwards.

The pain of acute cholecystitis comes on gradually so that most patients have had symptoms for about 48 hours before they come to hospital. During this time they will also have developed anorexia and nausea and may have vomited. They may have a raised temperature and 70 per cent of them will have had previous attacks – although probably not so severe. Nearly all the patients describe the pain as being on the right-hand side of the abdomen and almost half of them accurately localize it in the right upper quadrant. The pain is made worse by deep inspiration and if they also have right shoulder tip pain then the diagnosis is fairly certain. Jaundice is another confirmatory symptom which is present in about a quarter of all cases. On abdominal palpation there is tenderness in the right upper quadrant. Murphy's sign – pain accompanying inspiration on palpation under the right costal margin – is further strong evidence for the diagnosis. A straight X-ray of the abdomen will help to exclude other abdominal crises, such as small bowel obstruction and perforated duodenal ulcer, and may reveal a gall bladder full of stones.

Acute pancreatitis

This condition is seen in middle-aged men who regularly drink alcohol. It is sometimes associated with gallstone disease, usually in elderly female subjects. In other patients the condition is described as 'idiopathic' when there is neither a drink problem nor biliary disease.

In the acute presentation the pain comes on suddenly and is felt in the upper half of the abdomen. The severity can vary greatly from a vague, possibly intermittent pain to an overwhelming pain similar to that of a perforated duodenal ulcer. The patient with a perforation rarely vomits more than once, repeated vomiting is typical of acute pancreatitis.

A plain X-ray of the abdomen may reveal the presence of gallstones or calcification of the pancreas but it is the serum amylase estimation which confirms the diagnosis. A level below 500 iu/l makes the diagnosis unlikely, above 2000 iu/l the diagnosis is confirmed. Recently an amylase stick has been introduced for demonstrating a colour change caused by a raised urinary amylase. A negative result on testing the urine is usually reliable in excluding a diagnosis of pancreatitis; a positive result merits confirmation by estimating the serum amylase.

Renal colic

Severe renal colic is unmistakable. The pain is excruciating. The patient looks grey, sweats, and may roll on the floor in agony. The pain radiates from the loin to the pubic region, often to the penis and scrotum in the male or to the labia in the female. No other disease produces these symptoms. There is no abdominal tenderness or rigidity but palpation of the kidney is usually painful. Strangury is also sometimes present. These symptoms are usually due to a renal calculus making its way down the ureter. Sometimes the stone is held up at the pelvic brim and can be demonstrated on a straight X-ray of the abdomen. When the stone completes its journey to the bladder the colic will cease, but these patients merit subsequent investigation of the urinary tract to detect the presence of other stones or other chronic disease.

Ruptured ectopic gestation and salpingitis

A young women, who has recently missed a period, is carried into the Emergency Department looking ashen. There has been a sudden onset of abdominal pain and she may have vomited once. The pulse is weak and rapid and the blood pressure is low. There is generalized abdominal tenderness and the abdomen is doughy. She looks and is exsanguinated. She has a ruptured ectopic pregnancy with a massive haemoperitoneum. Although these patients look as though they are about to die they almost always respond favourably to blood transfusion and surgery.

Acute salpingitis, when it occurs, may mimic a less severe form of ruptured ectopic pregnancy. Vaginal examination will reveal a tender swollen fallopian tube. Arrangements should be made for a gynaecologist to undertake the necessary treatment.

Further reading

F. T. DE DOMBAL (1980). *Diagnosis of Acute Abdominal Pain.* Churchill Livingstone

Chapter 22

Paediatric emergencies

A very large part of the work of any Accident Department involves the treatment of children. Unfortunately, it is only in recent years that the special needs of children have been recognized and many departments are totally inadequate with respect to facilities for treating these young patients. Ideally, every department should have a waiting area set aside for children and their parents. Such an area will do much to reduce the tension affecting both the child, the parents and the other patients. It is important that the area can be supervised by nursing staff; if parents cannot see, or be seen by the nurses, they will not use the facility in case they may be overlooked. It is also important that the necessary priority can be given to children who begin to feel unwell after they have registered in the department.

As far as is practical, waiting should be kept to a minimum. Even if this is not always possible, a sympathetic word from a member of the staff is always appreciated and allows the parent to draw attention to any problems they may have, such as having to collect another child from school.

It is all too easy for the doctor dealing with large numbers of adult patients to forget that children need a different approach. The manner of the nursing staff towards children and their parents should be studied by the doctor, as it has much to offer. When the children appear to be 'difficult', the nursing staff are usually able to quieten them fairly easily by using a cheerful, though sympathetic, approach which, while allowing for the age of the child, accepts that the patient is an individual and not a passive object to be treated mechanically with minimal conversation.

After an injury, both child and parent are upset; the parent's anxiety communicates itself to the child, who is already in a strange situation and, as a result, the nervous child becomes unapproachable, frightened and clings to the mother in distress. A few minutes spent talking to the child will go far to persuading the child to co-operate.

As a general principle, every effort should be made to minimize the occasions which produce crying in children. If one child cries, others in the department tend to follow suit, even though they are not being treated in any way. Apart from the noise level, which can be very high if several children are crying at once, it is preferable that children should not be disturbed before they are seen otherwise their management becomes more difficult.

Some children cannot be consoled by any approach and scream whenever an attempt is made to examine or treat them. Frequently this arises from the parent's failing to help or control the child. The only satisfactory way to handle such a child is for a nurse to take over while the parent waits in another room.

Some children, far from being upset by the situation, appear to be thoroughly enjoying themselves. It is possible with these individuals to have a very pleasant conversation, during which the examination can be carried out without distress to either child or parent. Experience gained in handling this type of child can be applied to similar situations in the more nervous individual with a gain in the doctor's efficiency.

The parent should be allowed to accompany the child during the treatment, even if this involves suturing under local anaesthesia. The child who is having a general anaesthetic can be accompanied by the mother until the anaesthetic has been induced. Provided the parent is not over-possessive and liable to interfere with the treatment, or extremely nervous and considered to be unsuitable to be present, nothing but good can come from encouraging the parent to comfort the child during the treatment. External wounds can be sutured under local anaesthetic with as much ease as would be found with a general anaesthetic, provided the parents have been told beforehand what is going to be done and what attitude they should adopt during the procedure, but they must be told if at any time they should feel faint they must report this immediately.

Children may require restraint for the purpose of examination and for treatment if the procedure is in any way uncomfortable. For example, it is usually an easy matter to inspect the ear drums of children of any age, but the removal of a foreign body from the nose may be difficult because the child keeps withdrawing or moving his head. A small child should be wrapped in a blanket while he is gently laid on a firm couch. The pillow should be removed and the head gently restrained by a nurse. It is preferable if the mother can hold the child's hand through the blanket. Larger children should sit on their parent's knees with their feet held between their parent's thighs. One of the parent's hands holds the child round the chest, trapping his arms, and the other hand holds the child round the forehead in the required position.

If the child is uncontrollable, and the parents appear to be contributing to the situation, it is preferable to separate the child and the parents until the procedures have been completed. Alternatively, if a general anaesthetic will not be required and delay will not be prejudicial, the child can be given an oral dose of 5–20 mg diazepam syrup.

A good general principle in the department is always to question the reason why children should be crying. It is not possible to avoid some children showing distress, but proper handling, together with the use of suitable sedatives and local or general anaesthesia when appropriate, will do much to avoid the development of a fear of doctors and hospitals in the patient.

The injured child

Treatment of the injuries follows the standard principles used in adults, but the junior doctor should be aware of certain important differences which modify the management of the young patient:

1. Certain procedures require the administration of a general anaesthetic. This should always be used if the child is distressed or co-operation cannot be anticipated. Such procedures as the removal of a foreign body from the eye, ear or nose may require this approach and it is always preferable to administer a general anaesthetic rather than causing great distress to the patient. Intravenous anaesthetic agents, used for induction by an anaesthetist skilled in handling children, are painless, rapid in action and free from mental distress. A child who is pale, apprehensive and distressed before the procedure usually looks significantly improved on recovery from the anaesthetic.

2. Children tend to 'over-react' to illness or injury when compared with adults suffering from similar conditions. For example, children after head injuries frequently present in the department with pallor which is out of proportion to the degree of the injury. It is a safe assumption to make that any child showing such pallor will vomit profusely within a very short time. After vomiting and a short rest, the child appears completely recovered. Management depends on the overall assessment of the head injury.

   Similarly, children are very prone to develop convulsions after head injury. This apparently serious complication must be treated by intravenous use of an anticonvulsant drug, e.g.

2–10 mg diazepam followed by admission for observation. The prognosis is good in these cases and complications are unlikely to follow.

3. Children react very quickly to blood loss, whether from open wounds or concealed haemorrhage. It is important to realize that it is the percentage of the circulating blood and not the absolute amount lost that is significant. An adult can easily lose 500 ml from the circulation without any adverse effect, but a similar sized haemorrhage in a child with a blood volume of only 2 litres would show significant effects and require urgent replacement therapy. Therefore all haemorrhage from wounds, and particularly those of the scalp and face, should be dealt with expeditiously and the bleeding controlled by pressure, ligature or suture, depending on the circumstances.

When external haemorrhage from, for example, a wound or a tooth socket, does not stop with the appropriate measures, the possibility of a bleeding diathesis must be considered, and it may be necessary to seek the advice of the Paediatric Unit, who should also be asked for assistance if difficulties are encountered in setting up an intravenous drip on a very small child.

Concern over the physical well-being of the child should not blind the doctor to the importance of determining the cause of the accident. The prevention of accidents is an important part of the work of any unit and, without information about the causation, prevention is not possible.

The parents of a child who has been injured by a situation which should have been corrected or which, on hind-sight, can be seen to be dangerous, may well have a feeling of guilt. Time should be taken to reassure them, using a non-accusatory manner. The Medical Social Worker can supplement this advice or help by a home visit; alternatively, the Health Visiting Services could be asked to call. Health Visitors have an important part to play in accident prevention in children; they have a statutory duty to care for children under 5 years. Their acceptance by the parents enables them to visit the home after injury and, apart from giving relevant advice about the care of the child, allows accident prevention to be discussed in home surroundings.

It is easier to deal with accident prevention in the home when only one family is involved. Hazardous situations in schools, playgroups or other public places require the involvement of the local authorities and are referred preferably to the consultant in charge of the department for him to take up the matter with the appropriate branch of the local authority.

Few situations cause such distress in a department as the arrival of a seriously ill or dead child after an accident. Many of the points mentioned later under 'Sudden Infant Death Syndrome' (*see below*) are relevant to the care of the parents of these children. The degree of parental distress can be extreme and the greatest help is obtained by sending for the other parent or a near relative. The general practitioner can be asked to call on the family when the parents have returned home and, if necessary, the Medical Social Worker will be able to involve the Social Services Department if it appears that the incident will add further problems to a family already suffering from significant social disruption.

An adult who seriously injures or kills a child accidentally will be subjected to major stress, associated with strong feelings of guilt. This must not be overlooked in the desire to give attention to the child and his parents. Reassurance, explanation, sedation and the involvement of the general practitioner may be equally necessary, but it is important, from a legal point of view, that the person who caused the injury should be advised that, irrespective of his feelings or the cause of the accident, he should never indicate to the parents that the accident was his fault. To do so would prejudice any action that might be considered appropriate by his insurance company and might be used in a prosecution against him. Even though it may appear unsympathetic and go against everyone's natural inclination, it is preferable that the two groups be kept apart and conversation between them limited to the absolute minimum.

Sudden infant death syndrome (cot death)

The *sudden* and *unexpected* death of an infant or small child accounts for about 2000 deaths annually in the UK. The majority occur betwen 2 and 4 months of age and are commoner in: those in poorer socio-economic groups, the winter months, those who were pre-term at delivery, and twins.

The arrival of a dead or near dead infant in the Department, often at around 7 a.m. necessitates a logical approach.

1. The child should be admitted to the Department.
2. If the child is verifiably dead, resuscitation should not be started. If there are signs of life vigorous resuscitation should be instituted. A history should be obtained from one of the parents.

3. The distressed parents should be found a private room in which to wait and any accompanying children should be looked after by a suitable person.
4. The Paediatric Department *must* be informed.
5. Before breaking the news of death to the parents review carefully all the information.
6. Unless there is a history of illness or the parent's attitude is suspicious, inform them of the likely diagnosis.
7. Explain that as there is no obvious explanation for the child's death the Coroner has to be notified.
8. Explain that the Coroner's office will contact the parents later that day, either directly or through the local police to take a detailed statement of the events. Explain, also, that the Coroner will require a post-mortem examination to be carried out to try to determine the cause of death.
9. Do not attach blame.
10. Always allow the parents opportunity, in private, of seeing, holding and cuddling their baby. Before transportation to the mortuary ensure that the baby is dressed to look presentable and if the parents are required to make formal identification for the police or Coroner always send someone to accompany them.
11. Before the parents leave the Department:
    (a) *Check* that the general practitioner and/or Health Visitor are informed.
    (b) *Check* that if mother is lactating immediate advice is given on its suspension.
    (c) *Check* that suitable transport is available to take them home.
    (d) *Check* that the booklet *Information for Parents Following the Sudden and Unexpected Death of Their Baby* is offered.
    (e) *Check* that the Coroner's office has been informed.

Some form of later counselling for the parents is necessary either by the general practitioner or the hospital Paediatric Unit.

You will find this a distressing problem to deal with and you should take any opportunity to discuss it with your senior colleagues.

Child abuse

The role of the Casualty Officer is to identify those children who may have been abused, to take a clear history and to refer early to the Paediatric Department. The management of this condition is complex and time-consuming and involves not only the Social Services Department but may involve the police. It is relatively infrequent in a busy department but if unrecognized carries a high morbidity and a significant mortality.

Physical Abuse has been widely publicized. Suspicion is raised if the injury(ies) are inexplicable by the history, if they are of differing ages or are so severe as to make a single accident unlikely, e.g. fractured skull in an infant with retinal haemorrhage is virtually pathognomic of being shaken and hit against a solid object. Curious lesions raise the index of suspicion, e.g. cigarette burns, linear scalds, linear full thickness burns, linear bruising, bruised cheeks, bruising that 'fits' an open hand or closed fist, bilateral black eyes without basal skull fracture, torn frenulum of the lip and bite marks.

Deprivation is hard to quantify. Children may be deprived of love, warmth, food, security or protection from accident. They may be quiet and unresponsive with a dull flat effect. They may have little or no interest in their surroundings. They may be undernourished and dirty. The height and weight must be noted and plotted on the appropriate centile chart for comparison with the 'normal' population. Dietary enquiry may reveal the presence of 'food lies'; some parents say these children eat three Shredded Wheat–can you?

Sexual Abuse is commoner than you think. Most victims are young girls and most assailants are older men who are normally 'close' to the family. The abuse may take many forms, ranging from simple exposure ('flashing') to full sexual intercourse. The long-term psychological morbidity is very high if unrecognized and untreated. Great care must be taken with all children who present with perineal trauma, with or without vaginal bleeding. Careful inspection may reveal bruising or lacerations near the introitus or anus. Formal examination should be carried out with care and may require a general anaesthetic. Forensic swabs for semen may also be necessary. Clearly this examination is best done by an experienced doctor.

When discussing your findings with the parents, never be accusatory. It is too easy to be filled with righteous indignation. Try not to be hostile but be objective. Take a clear history and carefully note all the findings. One hallmark of child abuse is an inconsistent history. Well-kept notes and diagrams are invaluable in later evaluation.

Each district will have its own routine for dealing with child abuse and the junior doctor should adhere to it. If you are in doubt you should discuss it with senior colleagues or a senior member of the Paediatric Department.

Foreign bodies

The diagnosis of a 'foreign body' is usually straightforward when the area can be inspected directly. Similarly, radio-opaque objects do not present difficulties in confirmation, but many are either completely or partially radiolucent. When requesting an X-ray to demonstrate a foreign body, the nature of the object should be stated on the X-ray form. If the foreign body is thought to be unlikely to show clearly, it may be helpful to X-ray a similar foreign body on a comparable part of the patient's body. This may enable objects which would not otherwise be demonstrable on the film, because of soft tissue shadows, to be identified with a reasonable degree of certainty.

Foreign bodies in the eye

It may be possible to remove a foreign body from the eye using local anaesthetic and a cotton wool pledget on an orange stick. The child should be lying on a firm surface and wrapped in a blanket to prevent movement. If the foreign body is firmly embedded in the cornea, it is unlikely that it will be possible to remove it except with a needle and it is wise to obtain the help of the Eye Department staff.

Foreign bodies in the nose

Foreign bodies in the nose can usually be removed using topical anaesthesia. The child should be on a firm surface and wrapped in a blanket. Occasionally the foreign body can be gripped in forceps but firm, round objects, e.g. beads, cannot be gripped with nasal forceps. The forceps slip off the object and may drive it further back into the nasal passages. They must be removed by applying pressure from behind and pulling the object forwards. A curved dissector or a probe with the tip bent over is a suitable instrument for the purpose. If the object is situated well back and high up in the nose, the ENT Department should be consulted. If it cannot be removed easily or bleeding starts, referral is indicated. Indeed it is always wise to stop before bleeding is started by unskilled attempts at removal. Bleeding makes the task of the surgeon much more difficult and it is an axiom of work in the Accident and Emergency Department that the task of any doctor taking over a case from the unit shall not be made more difficult by unskilled or inappropriate management in the department.

If the foreign body has been in the nose for several days, it will be partly obscured by swelling of the tissues and a discharge, which is usually foul smelling. Peanuts may become very firmly impacted because they swell in the presence of moisture from the nasal secretions.

Foreign bodies in the ear

Foreign bodies in the external auditory meatus are technically difficult to remove because of the necessity to work through a speculum, using special instruments. The majority of children with these foreign bodies should be referred to the ENT Department. Syringing is not usually advisable. If the meatus is completely occluded, this would force the foreign body further in and might damage the drum. It is contraindicated in the presence of a perforation and further damage could be caused by movement of the child during the procedure. It should only be attempted with foreign bodies which are superficial and do not occlude the meatus. Minimal pressure is essential and the jet of water should be directed towards the gap above or at the side of the foreign body. The position of the foreign body must be checked frequently and the attempt stopped it it does not move. If the attempt is successful the meatus should be gently dried with cotton wool pledgets and the drum inspected to exclude damage.

Inhaled foreign bodies

Inhaled foreign bodies are associated with an attack of coughing and respiratory distress of a varying degree. If the distress persists, it suggests some degree of occlusion of the air passages.

The pharynx should be inspected with the child in the head-down position. If the foreign body can be seen to be near the larynx, removal should only be attempted if suitable instruments are available. If the foreign body becomes dislodged and occludes the larynx, a small child should promptly be held in the air by the feet and the back smacked. In older children an alternative is the Heimlich manoeuvre. The attendant stands behind the sitting child, places both arms around the abdomen as in a bear hug and sharply squeezes. This sudden rise in infradiaphragmatic pressure is transmitted upwards and is sufficient to expel the foreign body. The urgency of the situation is such that manual removal or dislodgement with a finger should be tried, otherwise tracheostomy may be required. This is technically very difficult in a young child with respiratory occlusion and it is advisable to avoid attempting any procedure which may result in this being necessary.

If it is thought that the object has entered one of the bronchi, an X-ray should be taken. Radio-opaque foreign bodies are clearly demonstrated but, unfortunately, many objects do not show directly on the film and their presence may have to be deduced by the development of changes in the lungs. If there is a strong probability of an inhaled foreign body being present based on the history and possibly on the presence of abnormalities in the breath sounds, the child should be referred to the ENT Department with a view to bronchoscopy.

When there is a possibility of a radiolucent foreign body, the chest should be re-X-rayed after 4 hours. Occlusion of a bronchus will produce collapse of the appropriate segment of the lungs.

No child should be discharged from medical supervision until the doctor is satisfied that the foreign body is not in the lungs. This may require further X-rays at weekly intervals until the absence of pulmonary changes confirms the absence of the foreign body, and it is always advisable to notify the general practitioner about the situation in case chest symptoms arise in the more remote future and the possibility of a foreign body may be overlooked if the information is not available.

All cases must be dealt with on their merits and, while most alleged inhaled foreign bodies have either been swallowed or coughed out, it is unsafe to assume that this occurred without taking steps to ensure that a negative initial assessment will not prejudice the child's future well-being.

Foreign bodies in the oesophagus

Foreign bodies impacted in the oesophagus give rise to difficulty in swallowing. Radiolucent foreign bodies cannot be seen on X-rays, but should be suspected if the child is unable to swallow water. The presence of such a foreign body can be confirmed by a barium swallow, using a minimal amount of contrast medium, but if the child is considered to need a contrast medium investigation, it is preferable to refer him to the ENT Department without further investigation.

Swallowed foreign bodies

Swallowed foreign bodies smaller in diameter than a 5 pence piece should pass through any child old enough to swallow such an object. If it can be clearly established that the foreign body is of such a size that it will pass through the child, there is little point in X-ray examination. The parents should be advised to allow the child a normal diet and not administer purgatives. The motions should be examined under water to see if the foreign body has been passed. Unless the child develops symptoms such as abdominal pain or vomiting, concern need not be felt if the foreign body is not found.

X-ray examination is advisable to detect the presence of sharp metallic objects, such as a pin, an open safety pin or a nail, or objects which might not pass through because of their size or shape. When X-ray shows a pin or similar pointed object, the child should be admitted in case the foreign body perforates the intestine. Objects which might not pass through have their progress studied in serial X-rays at daily or longer intervals until they have been excreted. If they do not progress through the alimentary tract, the child should be referred to the Surgical Unit in case laparotomy is necessary. The parents must be advised, if the child is being treated as an out-patient, to bring him or her back to the department immediately if abdominal pain or vomiting develops.

Poisoning

A safe assumption, when dealing with children, is that there is no solid or liquid substance which has properties that will inhibit a child from attempting to eat or drink it. Fortunately, in spite of their catholic tastes in this direction, the annual mortality remains low, but the number of children admitted to hospital for treatment or, more usually, for observation remains high. Household cleaning products are high on the list of substances, but drugs and medicines prescribed for the child, the parents, the grandparents or neighbours are one of the groups that cause concern. The other group of dangerous products is garden chemicals. These, for example paraquat, are highly toxic.

The Accident Officer should always be aware of his responsibility in the field of accident prevention by finding out how the child obtained the substance which has brought him to hospital and, if appropriate, make suggestions to the parents to avoid the situation recurring. The parents are frequently distressed after poisoning incidents and, if it is felt inappropriate at that time, the Health Visitor can be asked to make a home visit at a later date when advice may be more acceptable.

Management

The management of a case of poisoning in the Emergency Department involves:

1. The identification of the poison.
2. The treatment of any serious effects, e.g. convulsions or respiratory paralysis.
3. The elimination of the poison.
4. Admission to the Paediatric Department.

Identification of the poison

Identification may sometimes be a matter of informed guesswork, but usually the parents are sensible enough to bring a sample of the container to the hospital. Suitable tablet identification charts and reference books, which should be available in every department, are consulted to identify the precise nature of the chemical component, the specific treatment that may be needed and the various toxic effects that may arise. Reference can also be made to one of the Poisons Centres (*see* Appendix I) which hold comprehensive information about all the various aspects of drugs, chemicals and other products that are found within the home and in industry.

Estimation of the amount that the child may have consumed is also difficult. The majority of children spit the substance out without swallowing more than an insignificant amount but, when there is any possibility of a clinically significant consumption, a blood estimation should be carried out or, if appropriate, the laboratory should be asked to do a rapid screening test for some of the commoner drugs that are likely to be available to the child.

Blood estimations should always be carried out after the consumption of aspirin, barbiturates, psychotropic drugs, ferrous sulphate, paraquat and alcohol. Alcohol may produce significant hypoglycaemia and a blood sugar estimation should be done at the same time.

The time of consumption is important in relation to the development of symptoms and the necessity to carry out active treatment.

Initial treatment

Major adverse effects should be treated immediately. Respiratory depression takes precedence over all other aspects of the situation. The pharynx should be cleared by suction and an airway inserted, after which the child should be placed in the recovery position. Oxygen should be given through a face mask and, if these measures prove insufficient, assisted ventilation, using an Ambu bag or similar apparatus should be commenced. This can be followed by intubation and mechanical ventilation if the child does not make a very rapid improvement.

Convulsions should be controlled by intravenous diazepam: 0.25 mg/kg body weight up to 1 year of age; 2.5 mg between 1 and 7 years of age; 5 mg over 7 years of age.

Circulatory collapse with a systolic blood pressure below 100 mm Hg should be treated with an intravenous infusion of 5% glucose or normal glucose with one-fifth normal saline. Normal saline should not be used to avoid salt retention.

The Paediatric Department should always be consulted at an early stage when signs of toxicity are apparent, but urgent treatment must not be delayed while waiting for the arrival of either the paediatric or anaesthetic services.

Elimination of the poison

Most swallowed poisons are best treated by inducing vomiting with syrup of ipecacuanha: 10 ml from 6 to 18 months, and 15 ml if older. Half to one cup of water (or orange juice) should be given with the emetic. If vomiting does not occur within 20 minutes, the dose should be repeated. If vomiting does still not occur, it is essential that the stomach should be washed out to remove the emetic. The emetic should not be used if the patient is other than fully conscious, nor should vomiting be induced in kerosene or petrol poisoning because these substances are of greater danger if they contaminate the lungs than if they are left in the stomach.

Strong salt solutions are dangerous to use as emetics because of the risk of biochemical disturbances developing from the absorption of the sodium chloride.

Most drugs are absorbed or leave the stomach within 2 to 3 hours and there is little point in inducing vomiting after this time. Aspirin and ferrous sulphate are unusual because significant quantities can be recovered even after periods of 6 to 8 hours and it is well worthwhile to induce vomiting even after this time.

Tricyclic antidepressants rapidly cause ileus and may be

recovered after many hours, but they should be removed by gastric lavage as ipecacuanha is unlikely to work.

When removal of the drug is considered essential and the patient is unconscious, the air passages should be protected by a cuffed endotracheal tube before lavage is commenced. Water is an effective solution to use for this purpose and the procedure should be continued until the returns are clear. The head-down position must be used and every care taken to safeguard the respiratory tract. The mouth should be sucked clear at the end of the procedure and, if there is any doubt about the ability of the child to maintain a clear airway, the tube should be left in place.

The stomach contents should be preserved for laboratory investigation if the child presents the slightest sign of toxic effects or if the substance consumed cannot be identified.

Admission

Admission should always follow treatment in the Emergency Department. In most cases the child will not show any ill effects from the drug or chemical and observation for longer than 6 to 8 hours will not be necessary. The parents should be informed about the child's condition and the reason for admission, but it should be made clear that the responsibility for treatment has been handed over to the paediatric service.

Some specific poisons

Aspirin poisoning

Confirmation that the child has taken this drug can be obtained by the use of 'phenistix', which turns a deep purple colour when dipped in the child's urine.

Blood levels should be ascertained if the child is vomiting or hyperventilating. The drug produces a metabolic acidosis with a respiratory alkalosis, and blood gas and pH estimations are necessary for treatment after the stomach contents have been removed. Treatment is carried out by the Paediatric Department.

Iron preparations

These highly toxic drugs are frequently taken by children who swallow tablets that have been prescribed for their mothers and which have been left lying around the home. Vomiting is an early symptom. Gastric erosions may cause haematemesis and shock.

Prompt treatment is essential. Vomiting should be induced with ipecacuanha and the stomach should then be washed out using 2 g desferrioxamine in 1 litre of water; 10 mg desferrioxamine in 50 ml of water should be left in the stomach.

A blood sample should be sent to the laboratory to provide a primary level of the free iron content of the plasma, prior to the decision on the use of systemic desferrioxamine.

Paracetamol

Ipecacuanha should be used to produce vomiting. The blood paracetamol concentration should be measured at least *4 hours* after ingestion and the decision to treat with N-acetylcysteine should be made by the paediatricians.

The phenothiazines and tricyclic antidepressants

Large amounts of these drugs are in use among the population and consumption of a parent's capsules is not infrequent. The former are less toxic than the latter, but they can both cause disturbances of consciousness and respiratory depression.

Treatment follows standard practice but it should be noted that both can give rise to cardiac arrythmias. The patient should be carefully monitored on a cardioscope and the Paediatric Department contacted immediately if arrhythmias appear. Admission is essential, even if the amount consumed appears to be minimal.

Household products

There are vast numbers of proprietary products found in every house, garage, greenhouse or other outbuilding. These may include industrial products brought home by a parent for a particular purpose, e.g. dry cleaning clothes. They may contain petroleum products, corrosives and various complex and possibly toxic chemicals. Respiratory and circulatory depression must be treated immediately, but no attempt to induce vomiting or wash out the stomach should be made until the nature of the substances consumed has been established. The Poisons Information Centres have been provided with details of the formulation of most of the commoner proprietary preparations (e.g. metal cleaners, paints, polishes, etc.) on a confidential basis for use in treating patients, and they should be consulted whenever there is doubt about either the nature of the substance or the treatment necessary. Help may also be obtained locally from schools, colleges or firms in the neighbourhood and from time to time it may be necessary to consult the manufacturers of the particular product. The fire brigade also keeps a comprehensive index of industrial chemicals which are transported by road or which can be produced in fires, and the local College of Agriculture may be of assistance in the identification of plants, seeds or other vegetable products.

Other medical emergencies

Convulsions

One of the commonest paediatric emergencies is a young child suffering from convulsions. He is usually brought in at high speed by a very distressed mother. It is important to find out if the child has suffered from fits or blackouts, if he or she is receiving any medication and if there is a history of an injury or a febrile or other illness during the previous few days.

The convulsions must be controlled immediately. Up to 10 mg diazepam (depending on the child's age) should be given slowly intravenously. An airway is inserted, the pharynx cleared with a sucker and the child nursed in the recovery position.

The Paediatric Department should be notified of any case of convulsions in the Emergency Department, as the child will require admission. If the convulsions do not cease within 10 minutes, the Anaesthetic Department should be consulted because of the risk to the child of asphyxia, inhalation of vomit, permanent neurological deficiencies or even death. Status epilepticus, the condition in which the convulsions do not cease spontaneously or following treatment, may necessitate the induction of general anaesthesia and the use of muscle relaxants to enable a mechanical ventilator to be used until the fits have been brought under control.

The commonest cause of convulsions in children under the age of 5 years is a fever. Certain children, and often siblings, appear to have a genetic predisposition to react in this way. The cause of the fever may be an upper respiratory infection with or without otitis media. Apart from the use of anticonvulsive drugs, the child's temperature should be lowered by exposure, tepid sponging, and an aspirin suppository.

Fits may recur in the future if the child suffers a febrile illness, and it may be advisable to administer anticonvulsants on these occasions.

The parents should be reassured that one or two attacks of this nature are not due to epilepsy and that this response to a raised body temperature will probably cease by the time the child is 5 or 6 years of age.

Respiratory emergencies

Respiratory emergencies are properly the responsibility of the paediatric services. However, from time to time children are admitted with acute respiratory embarrassment which demands immediate attention in the Accident and Emergency Department.

Acute asthma

Status asthmaticus may develop suddenly during the night in an asthmatic child who has developed a minor respiratory infection. The clinical picture is one of marked cyanosis, over-action of the accessory muscles of respiration, retraction of the sternum and intercostal spaces, and obvious great distress in the child. The parents are very upset and the nursing staff are deeply concerned. The doctor should, if necessary, try and reduce the tension by reassuring the child and parents.

Oxygen should be administered – if this can be given through an efficient humidifier it will be of greater benefit.

Nebulised salbutamol or terbutaline often produces temporary relief; failing this, aminophylline (5 mg/kg body weight) given intravenously over 30 minutes may be effective. Caution must be exercised in the dose of aminophylline if the child is receiving a slow-release theophylline preparation as maintenance prophylaxis. Hydrocortisone (100 mg intravenously) should always be given. Failure to respond within 20 minutes requires urgent paediatric consultation.

Croup

Croup is the term used to describe the noisy respiration that children make with upper respiratory tract obstruction. Some of these conditions are potentially lethal. Urgent appraisal is therefore necessary.

Acute epiglottitis (Supraglottitis)

This is an acute inflammation of the larynx and supraglottic structures. It is usually seen in children between 2 and 5 years of age and is usually caused by *Haemophilus influenzae* type B. Fortunately it is uncommon but if inappropriately managed leads to acute respiratory tract obstruction and death in 50 per cent of patients.

The condition usually presents as progressively noisy breathing. The noise made is often expiratory as well as inspiratory. True 'barking' stridor is rare and if it occurs usually indicates laryngotracheobronchitis (*see* below). The child is ill, frightened, often cyanosed and has marked respiratory distress. Dysphagia is characteristic, the child being unable to swallow even his own saliva and thus he drools.

Having made this diagnosis *urgent* paediatric and experienced anaesthetic help is required. No investigations should be carried out until help is to hand; the slightest noxious stimulus may be sufficient to precipitate acute airways obstruction. The child must be observed closely; if airways obstruction occurs then endotracheal intubation is indicated using the oral route. Tracheostomy done under these circumstances is not the treatment of choice.

Acute laryngotracheobronchitis (Infraglottitis)

This is much commoner than epiglottitis. It is usually viral in origin, presenting often in the early hours of the morning. Characteristically the child is well during the day, goes to bed normally and awakens with a barking cough and inspiratory stridor. The age range is usually 1–3 years. Often the stridor has subsided by the time the child has reached Casualty (possibly a function of the outside temperature). He is not ill, usually bright and alert, not cyanosed but may have a barking cough with distress. He can drink a cup of squash or water. Admission is necessary to observe and ensure that the distress does not increase.

Gastroenteritis

It is not uncommon for parents whose children are suffering from gastroenteritis of infancy to by-pass their general practitioner and bring the child straight to the Emergency Department.

Dehydration is the principle medical indication for admission. Skin turgor should be assessed as should the state of the oral mucous membranes. Severe dehydration (more than 10 per cent of the expected body weight) is associated with a dry mouth, sunken eyes, listlessness and hypovolaemia. Paediatric advice is clearly indicated. Mild dehydration can be managed with cessation of normal diet and the use of oral rehydration solutions, glucose/electrolyte mixtures (GEM).

Chapter 23

Medical emergencies

The management of a medical emergency arriving unexpectedly in a department fully occupied with the treatment of a large number of traumatic cases presents the inexperienced junior doctor with many problems. In contrast to patients in out-patient departments, a good history may be difficult to obtain. The patient is frightened, distressed, confused or, in many cases, unconscious. It is unusual to obtain an accurate history of previous illnesses or conditions for which the patient is currently being treated by his general practitioner and personal information in a handbag or wallet may be sufficient to enable a relative or the patient's practitioner to be contacted.

The Emergency Department has four functions in the management of a medical emergency, and it is important that the doctor realizes the limitations imposed on his clinical management because of the circumstances that exist in these units. The doctor should follow standard routine when dealing with any unexpected medical emergency–he should avoid making 'spot' diagnoses and should try and avoid being rushed into making decisions before he has had time to consider, and if necessary discuss, the appropriate management of the patient. It is easy in the busy atmosphere of an Emergency Department to make errors of judgement. Many such errors do not affect the well-being of the patient in any way, but it is difficult to defend errors such as sending patients home when they live on their own and are not physically fit to care for themselves. A study of the newspaper columns will produce other examples and remind the doctor of the vulnerable position he holds. If in doubt, he should always play it safe.

The management of a medical emergency

Immediate emergency care

When appropriate, the first step should always be the establishment of a clear airway. Noisy breathing means airway obstruction. This may be caused by the tongue or by vomit or both. The obstruction should be relieved by positioning, the insertion of an airway, clearing the pharynx by suction and, if all else fails, intubation should be carried out and a cuffed endotracheal tube inserted.

Cyanosis will require the administration of oxygen by face mask or through a rebreathing bag connected to an endotracheal tube if the simpler method is inadequate and the patient is unconscious. If there is marked depression of the rate and depth of respiration, manual assisted ventilation should be used. Oxygen concentrations of more than 30 per cent should not be given to patients with cyanosis who are suffering from carbon dioxide retention as, for example, in emphysema. The patient's respiratory centre is depressed by the high level of carbon dioxide and breathing is being stimulated solely by the hypoxia; if the hypoxia is abolished by oxygen in high concentration the respiratory drive will be abolished.

Diagnosis

Once the airway has been dealt with, the doctor can obtain any history that is available. Frequently this amounts to no more than the fact that the patient collapsed in a street or in a shop. Some patients have been found collapsed in their home, where they may have been lying on the floor for prolonged periods; others may be brought in from work. Information on these patients may be obtained from the works medical or home nursing services. Information about school children can be obtained from the school or a teacher who has accompanied the child to hospital.

The simultaneous arrival of several patients who are members of a group suggests a common factor in the disorder, e.g. food poisoning or exposure to toxic fumes.

The ambulance attendants can give details of the circumstances under which the patient was found. They may bring in tablets or tablet containers found near the patient. Further information may be obtained by searching the patient's clothes. Tablets, the address of relatives, the name of the practitioner and other useful information may be found.

Examination follows normal clinical practice. The patient's temperature should be taken with a low-reading thermometer to avoid missing hypothermia.

The respiratory rate may be greatly modified by various disorders. For example, it will be increased in hyperventilation tetany and may be of a Cheyne-Stokes character in cerebral haemorrhage. Barbiturate overdose with cyanosis and depression of respiration has become less frequent due to the diminished use of barbiturates by general practitioners.

Irregularities in the pulse may indicate fibrillation as a possible source of embolic phenomena. A slow pulse will be found in heart block, cerebral haemorrhage or hypothermia. An increased pulse rate may indicate haemorrhagic or cardiovascular shock or, in the conscious patient, it may only be a manifestation of alarm at being involved in an unfamiliar situation. Significant changes in the blood pressure at the upper and lower end of the scale can provide pointers to the diagnosis.

Much can be learnt by watching the patient. Disturbances in consciousness, dyspnoea and neurological abnormalities can be assessed rapidly and easily in this manner. A restless patient may be shocked, or hypoxic, or hypoglycaemic.

Large numbers of bruises in the elderly usually suggest sub-optimal nutrition in a person living on his own. If the patient's name and address is known, information might be available from the Social Services Department.

Examination should be rapid and should cover all systems. Inspection of the fundi should not be forgotten.

The urine should be examined, if necessary after catheterization.

Biochemical investigations may be required as a matter of urgency. Blood sugar levels can be checked rapidly with Dextrostix, while awaiting results from the laboratory. Blood gas analysis may be necessary in respiratory or biochemical disorders. The laboratory may also be required to carry out a screening of the blood when poisoning is suspected with paracetamol, salicylates, or iron.

If the patient smells of alcohol, it does not necessarily mean that the patient is drunk. This is a well recognized clinical trap. When the level of alcohol is of clinical importance, a blood sample should be taken for immediate analysis.

X-ray examination is of value in the acute medical situation. Chest X-rays may reveal pathology; skull X-rays may show a shift in the position of the pineal body and, from time to time, both chest and skull X-rays may show evidence of a systemic disease, e.g. secondary carcinomatosis or myeloma.

Electrocardiography is essential when cardiac disease is suspected. A definite abnormality is helpful, but unfortunately a normal tracing does not exclude disease. Infarction abnormalities may not develop for several hours and early confirmation of this condition may best be obtained by changes in the enzyme levels.

Treatment

Treatment should normally be limited to the minimum necessary to provide good clinical care of the patient. An Emergency Department is not the appropriate area in which to carry out detailed investigation or to initiate complex therapeutic measures. The patient will only be in the department for a short time before being admitted or discharged home and any measures used must be limited to the immediate requirements of the situation. Nevertheless, if there is proper liaison between the intaking medical firm and the Emergency Department, definitive treatment can in some cases be started before the patient is sent to the ward.

Patients who are sent home should always be provided with a letter informing their general practitioner about the treatment that they were given in the unit. A period of observation after treatment is a wise precaution, particularly for elderly patients, even if the only treatment required was a cup of tea.

Disposal

Correct disposal of a patient is a much more important matter than many juniors assume it to be when they start to work in an Emergency Department. The patient will be admitted to the wards in either the hospital to which he was taken or to those in a neighbouring hospital. He will be discharged to his home or that of a relative or friend, to a local authority institution or into the care of the police.

Frequently the distances involved may be considerable and transport by car or ambulance may be necessary. If relatives have not accompanied the patient to hospital, they must always be advised as to which hospital the patient has been admitted.

If the patient's condition is poor and transfer is unavoidable, then a nurse or doctor should accompany him, taking with them equipment that might be needed on the journey. Suitable apparatus for this purpose should always be readily available and should include intubation and oxygen equipment, a battery-operated cardioscope and defibrillator, and appropriate drugs for dealing with cardiac arrest or infusion therapy. The journey should be slow and steady. If a high speed journey with horns blaring, lights flashing and police escort is considered necessary, it is probable that the patient is unfit for the transfer.

Many patients are discharged home only after considerable thought. The chronic bed shortage may mean that some are sent home who would, under ideal conditions, be admitted. This unhappy situation places an added burden on the doctor, who must take steps to ensure that appropriate arrangements have been made for the patient's well-being after discharge. The patient who can go home and be looked after by a relative or friend is fortunate. It is only necessary to establish that the circumstances are adequate to provide the appropriate care, i.e. a frail elderly lady cannot hope to deal with a large bedridden elderly man. The Medical Social Worker should be asked to investigate the home situation before the patient is moved from the hospital and they may be able to arrange community-based support services.

When one member of an elderly infirm couple is taken to hospital and admission is not considered necessary, the Medical Social Worker may be able to arrange for help to be provided which will make home care of the patient a practical proposition. Such help may include relatives or neighbours. Alternatively, a home help may be provided by the local authority. The District Nurse may be asked to call and the meals on wheels service can be asked to help in providing meals of adequate quality at least once a day. In some areas the hospital authorities are introducing a twilight nursing service, which will enable nursing care to be made available for a greatly extended period during the evening and part of the night. These measures enable many patients, who would otherwise be admitted to hospital, to be cared for in the community. The general practitioner should always be informed by letter or telephone.

The patient who lives on his own may be able to manage if similar arrangements can be made for his discharge, but it is obvious that even more care should be taken that all the necessary arrangements have been made for the patient's continuing support. Sometimes patients who live on their own can be admitted to local authority hostels. These hostels only provide 'hotel facilities' and patients who are unable to dress or move about freely probably cannot be accommodated.

Cardiac arrest

The patient is usually presented to the receiving doctor in the back of an ambulance having been telephoned in as a collapse, presumably due to cardiac arrest. The fact that the ambulance personnel have brought the patient and have performed CPR on the way to hospital means that the circumstances suggested either the presence of signs of life when first seen, or a short enough history to allow hope of resuscitation. This judgment needs generally to be accepted, and a further attempt made by the Casualty staff even though there seems little hope.

The following steps are carried out:

1. Feel for a pulse, carotid or femoral. Also note swiftly the pupils, the skin colour and temperature, and confirm the absence of respiration. If arrest is confirmed . . .
2. Thump the sternum once, firmly.
3. Commence external cardiac massage.
4. Clear the airway.
5. Establish ventilation via a mask or endotracheal tube.
6. Cannulate a vein, and correct acidosis.
7. Obtain electrocardiograph monitoring and treat accordingly.

Two things are immediately evident. First, the back of an ambulance is not a suitable place for CPR and the patient should quickly be transferred to the resuscitation area on a firm trolley. Secondly, it is difficult for a doctor to perform CPR alone, and with help the above steps will be concurrent not consecutive.

External cardiac massage (ECM)

If there is a stop-clock in the resuscitation room this should be routinely started when the patient is brought in.

A firm surface is essential, and it must be possible for the operator to be high enough to be able to push down on the sternum with shoulders directly over the chest. If the blow to the chest is not successful, compression should be commenced 60 times a minute. The downward thrust must be forceful, with the heel of both hands, one on the other, over the lower one-third of the sternum in the mid-line.

The emphysematous chest may be impossible to compress without fracturing the costal cartilages. A child on the other hand will require proportionately less force.

Adequacy of the cardiac compression must be checked by arterial pulsations in the groin or neck.

Airway and ventilation

Patients arriving at the emergency entrance with cardiac standstill have usually been subjected to adequately performed ECM. Ventilation has, however, often been neglected. Immediate airway clearance and positive pressure oxygenation is necessary.

Suction is ideal, but false teeth and gross vomitus can be removed with a guarded finger and mouth to mouth ventilation begun as a basic measure. A Brook airway is useful at this stage but a bag and mask such as an Ambu bag is more efficient and should be used until endotracheal intubation can be performed and ventilation carried out with 100 per cent oxygen.

For endotracheal intubation choose for an average adult a 8.5–9.5 mm cuffed tube, but for the child choose an uncuffed tube appropriate to its age (*see* Appendix II—Paediatric Data) or one that approximates to the diameter of the child's little finger. An introducer should be available if required.

After introduction of the tube, inflate the cuff, attach a bag and watch the chest move with compression of the bag, or auscultate, to ensure the tube is correctly placed. This technique of intubation must be practised on a mannikin or cadaver. All the equipment used must be familiar and in particular the paediatric resuscitation kit must be separately packed and clearly labelled for immediate access.

Ventilate the patient at 10–15 times per minute. It is not necessary to phase this to fit in with the cardiac massage, but both should be simultaneously performed with independent rhythms.

Intravenous access (*see* Chapter 25)

While ECM and oxygenation are being established another member of the team should insert a large cannula with an injection port into any available vein. If a large antecubital vein can be cannulated a long catheter is introduced to monitor the central venous pressure.

100 mmol of sodium bicarbonate solution (100 ml of 8.4%) is given immediately as a bolus. The line is cleared with saline and 0.5 g of calcium gluconate is given in a 10 ml solution.

If there is difficulty obtaining a vein, subclavian or internal jugular vein cannulation should be attempted, or if experience in this is lacking an immediate cut-down procedure should be used.

Diagnosis

Electrocardiograph monitoring will probably have been initiated by this time by the nursing staff, but if not, should be performed through defibrillator paddles. The diagnosis can then be made and the appropriate further steps initiated.

Asystole

This is the commonest finding in Accident and Emergency practice and represents too often the end stage. Both atropine (2 mg i.v.)

and adrenaline (10 ml of 1:10 000 i.v. or down the endotracheal tube) are used and if there is any doubt about the efficiency of cardiac massage or any difficulty obtaining venous access they should be given by the intracardiac route, through the fourth left intercostal space immediately lateral to the sternum, or from beneath the costal margin adjacent to the xiphoid cartilage.

One of three things will happen. If sinus rhythm ensues and remains no further measures are taken. If ventricular fibrillation is induced it is managed as detailed below. If there is no response CPR is continued, and further boluses of adrenaline (or isoprenaline 100 µg) are used. Pacemaker insertion via oesophagus, transthoracic or transvenous route is considered. This decision would normally be taken by a coronary care team. If there is no response after 30 minutes of efficient CPR the attempt can be abandoned.

Ventricular fibrillation

The defibrillator is charged to 200 joules while CPR is continuing, and the shock given across the heart, one paddle to the right of the sternum and the other held to the left-hand side of the chest behind the anterior axillary line. If there is no response, further shocks are tried with energy levels increasing by 100 joules each time to a maximum of 400 joules. CPR must be continued consistently between times. If there is still no response, 100 mg lignocaine is given as a bolus intravenously and the shock repeated. If there is still no response the blood gases and electrolytes should be checked and specialist help sought with regard to alternative drug therapy. At no time should CPR be stopped until such a decision is formally made.

Other dysrhythmias

A number of dysrhythmias are seen during resuscitation, and they should call for management by a specialist team. For example, ventricular tachycardia will also require cardioversion if carotid sinus massage or drugs are ineffective.

Electromechanical dissociation

The clinical picture is of complexes without detectable cardiac output. Look for the raised CVP of cardiac tamponade, and remember pneumothorax with tension. Also, check history for drugs.

An x-ray examination of the chest would show the cardiomegaly of tamponade, and the hilar prominence of massive pulmonary embolism.

If these can all be excluded, treat with adrenaline, or isoprenaline, repeated if necessary, and give calcium chloride 0.5 G i.v.

Breaking bad news (*see* Chapter 2, p. 15)

Any accompanying relatives must be kept in touch with what is happening. This will be done in the main by a nurse who will stay with them in a suitable room, but news of the outcome must be communicated, with the utmost sensitivity, by the doctor. If the relative telephones, the identity and relationship must be known before serious or confidential information is given.

Pain in the chest

Any patient who presents with chest pain must be assessed immediately, and if cardiogenic pain is a possibility further investigation is best done in the resuscitation area. An intravenous cannula is inserted into the back of the hand and a cardiac monitor applied. Intravenous diamorphine and intramuscular Stemetil (12.5 mg) are injected to give pain relief. Care will need to be exercised not to miss the unusual presentation with back pain, pain in the shoulder or arm, or even abdominal pain. An ECG and enzyme studies may be normal but, on the history alone, if cardiogenic pain is suspected specialist advice should be sought before sanctioning discharge.

Acute dyspnoea

It is usually clear whether the dyspnoea is due to a cardiorespiratory or a metabolic cause. Airway obstruction is also distinctive. It is crucial to obtain as much information from relations, or work-mates, as possible.

Pulmonary oedema

The patient is sitting up, coughing, sometimes wheezing. Distress is profound and clinical shock is present with central cyanosis. Basal crepitations may be present and basal congestion is evident on X-ray. ECG examination will probably reveal the cause, whether ischaemia or arrhythmia. Blood gases also supply useful information.

Management

1. Give intravenous morphine; begin with 2.5 mg and increase the dose according to the response.
2. Support the patient as upright as possible and give high oxygen flow through a face mask. If there is known obstructive airways disease care should be taken not to reduce the respiratory drive.
3. Give aminophylline 250 mg intravenously slowly, unless an arrhythmia is present.
4. Give frusemide 80 mg intravenously over 5 minutes.
5. If respiratory failure supervenes, bronchoscopy and bronchial toilet, and endotracheal intubation with assisted ventilation will be required.

Asthma

A patient who has had previous attacks and is under treatment is only likely to attend if the asthma is out of control, unless he has run out of his inhalant at the weekend, or is away from home. It may not be realized at first how ill this patient is, and the following serve as important guidelines:

1. The patient who is distressed knows his own condition well and his concern needs to be acted on.
2. Tachycardia of greater than 120 per minute, cyanosis, poor chest wall excursion and little wheezing all signify a serious attack.
3. The peak-flow meter is used to quantify the attack. The normal peak flow rate is over 400 L/min, and if the result is less than 100 L/min the patient is severely ill.
4. Exhaustion and diminished conscious level are ominous signs.

Management

1. Give oxygen through a nebulizer containing 0.5% salbutamol.
2. Cannulate a vein and give:

   (i) intravenous aminophylline 250 mg (average adult) over 5–10 minutes.
   (ii) 100 mg hydrocortisone intravenously.
3. Alert the specialist team immediately.
4. X-ray the chest. Watch out for pneumothorax.

5. Measure blood gases.
6. The patient may need assisted ventilation if tachycardia over 120/min persists, the P_{O_2} remains less than 5 kPa, the P_{CO_2} rises, and the patient becomes dehydrated and exhausted.

Pneumothorax

Unilateral chest pain with varying degrees of dyspnoea in a young man is typical of the spontaneous variety, and rarely causes much distress. The less common variety in obstructive airways disease causes alarm out of all proportion to its size and can constitute a life-threatening emergency. The traumatic variety is dealt with in Chapter 7 (*see* p. 51).

An expiratory chest film highlights the collapsed lung edge. Tension is evidenced by displacement of the mediastinal structures.

Management

If dyspnoea is present, intercostal drainage is appropriate (*see* Chapter 25), but this is a considered procedure and the emergency cannulation of the pleural space is required only if tension is considerable.

Hyperventilation

When the patient is seen, characteristic overbreathing may not be obvious, but the complaint will usually be of tingling in hands and feet, and a feeling of spasm in the muscles of the face and hands. Anxiety is often present, and an alteration of conscious level may be noted. Examination is unremarkable except for main d'accoucheur, and rebreathing from a paper bag will solve the problem.

If any doubt exists, arterial pH and blood gases are measured and alkalosis with a raised P_{O_2} are found.

Pulmonary embolism

The patient with massive embolisation is usually brought in having collapsed and presents the features of terminal cardiogenic shock, or cardiac arrest. The diagnosis is then made by post-mortem.

However, the patient may be conscious enough to complain of severe central chest pain, and is acutely dyspnoeic, with central cyanosis unless profoundly shocked, hypotension and tachycardia. The jugular venous pressure is increased and the patient may be less distressed lying down than sitting up.

If a history is obtained, a recent operation, or period of immobilization is relevant. X-ray examination shows increased hilar markings. The ECG may be normal but classically shows an S wave in lead I, a Q and an inverted T wave in lead III. Arterial blood gas estimation is done immediately and shows a low P_{O_2} level.

Management

Give oxygen, and employ external cardiac massage if the output is failing. Insert an intravenous cannula and give 15 000 units of heparin. Full CPR may, of course, be needed from the beginning.

Further anticoagulation, and more sophisticated investigations of the lung fields will depend on the immediate outcome and will be initiated by the specialist team if the patient survives the initial event.

Pulmonary infarct

The patient who presents with chest pain of pleuritic type and blood-stained sputum may also be dyspnoeic and distressed. A pleural rub may be heard in the area of the pain, but X-ray frequently does not show localized shadowing. The ECG is unhelpful but the white cell count is frequently raised.

Any previous incident should be specifically asked about and any existing signs of peripheral deep vein thrombosis noted.

The treatment will be to anticoagulate, but unless the patient's condition is exceptionally urgent this should be left to the admitting team.

Metabolic dyspnoea

The lack of respiratory distress is characteristic. The cause may be salicylate overdosage or diabetic ketoacidosis, or renal or hepatic failure. The management is that of the cause.

Diabetes

Hyperglycaemia

A patient with known diabetes under therapy may present with ketoacidosis as a result of intercurrent infection or illness, or perversity. The diagnosis is rarely difficult but coma can develop rapidly and urgent management by the specialist team is required.

The patient who presents in pre-coma or coma with previously undiagnosed diabetes has had polyuria, thirst, and increasing lassitude and malaise over several days at least. This sometimes has been misinterpreted by relatives and the family doctor, and the subject may arrive seriously ill, or with apparently irrelevant symptoms such as abdominal pain.

Dextrostix examination of the blood, or urine testing, will give immediate confirmation and intravenous normal saline is begun immediately. The patient may well vomit and a nasogastric tube should be inserted. No attempt should be made initially to give large amounts of water by mouth.

Hypoglycaemia

Although most patients recognize the gradual onset of symptoms and are able to take appropriate action, the onset of hypoglycaemia can be sufficiently sudden to catch out even careful patients. The diagnosis must be considered in any case of collapse, and evidence of diabetic therapy sought from the patient's possessions, or from the relatives.

The features are as follows: a rapid onset of unusual behaviour, confusion, often aggression, with increasing drowsiness, sweating, tachycardia, pallor, and occasionally various neurological signs including fits or hemiparesis. An immediate Dextrostix reading provides the answer, and 50 ml of 50% dextrose solution is injected through a large bore needle into a substantial vein in the antecubital fossa.

Recovery is dramatic, but care should be taken if a long-acting insulin is responsible and he should be admitted either for short-term observation and food by mouth, or for longer-term stabilization.

Routine urine testing

Many previously undiagnosed patients are discovered in Accident and Emergency departments through routine testing of the urine. This is particularly relevant where there is local sepsis, such as an abscess, or evidence of peripheral vascular disease or problems with vision.

Loss of consciousness

The onset may be sudden or gradual and the episode may be short-lived or be persisting when the patient arrives. An accurate history is therefore vital and every available witness must be canvassed, including ambulance personnel, relatives, bystanders, shop assistants, etc.

If a head injury or oligaemic shock can be excluded, a brief assessment is usually able to distinguish between the commoner causes. The procedure should be as follows:

1. Secure the airway if unconsciousness persists.
2. Make sure ventilation is adequate, if necessary using a spirometer to measure minute volume. Note the characteristics of the respiration.
3. Record the pulse, blood pressure and peripheral perfusion.
4. Note any breath odours such as alcohol, ketones or uraemic foetor.
5. Check the conscious level using the Glasgow Coma Scale (see Chapter 4), and examine for neck stiffness, pupillary and fundal changes, and note the muscle tone and peripheral reflexes.
6. Note the rectal temperature, if necessary using a low-reading thermometer.
7. Search for needle puncture marks, and for any evidence of drug bottles, notes, and of course any relevant previous medical history such as steroid and diabetic cards.

If the patient is conscious but gives a history of unconsciousness or collapse, it is usually possible to distinguish between a 'fit' or a 'faint', i.e. between a neurological and a cardiovascular cause. The witness may give a clear picture of an epileptiform seizure, or the patient may describe a vasovagal syncope. It may have been a transient ischaemic, or 'drop' attack without loss of consciousness, or it may have been a Stokes-Adams episode and there may be pronounced bradycardia in a conscious patient when seen. The patient with the common syncopal episode usually is sent home, and the patient with epilepsy also, unless status is threatened or it is a first attack. However where ECG abnormalities exist further in-patient investigation is indicated.

If the patient is still unconscious, or the conscious level is disturbed, the diagnosis will commonly rest between some form of cerebrovascular incident, hypoglycaemia, drug overdosage (including alcohol) and status epilepticus. Less common causes will include diabetic coma, hepatic or renal failure, meningitis, CO_2 narcosis and hysteria.

Cerebrovascular causes

These will usually be a bleed or infarct in an elderly person with deep unconsciousness and focal signs of hemiparesis together with hypertension. However an important diagnosis is the subarachnoid haemorrhage in a younger patient with a history from the relative of a premonitory headache followed by a sudden loss of consciousness. Neck stiffness is present and the presence of blood in the spinal fluid confirms the diagnosis. The patient is referred urgently to the neurosurgical unit for CT scan, care being taken to maintain a clear airway and satisfactory ventilation meanwhile.

Hypoglycaemia

This has been referred to above (*see* p. 190)

Drug overdosage

This may provide certain characteristic clinical pictures. Alcohol is betrayed on the breath and can be accurately estimated in breath or blood. Care, however, should be taken to exclude other drugs or a head injury. Opiates depress the respiration and the pin-point pupils and altered conscious level rapidly respond to naloxone. *Barbiturates* produce profound coma and hypotension and the drug can be estimated in the serum. *Carbon monoxide* is suspected by the circumstances in which the patient is found and although the classic cherry-red mucosae are not always obvious, arterial blood gas estimation, and carboxyhaemoglobulin levels confirm the diagnosis. Cardiac arrhythmias and profound hypotension may be present and high concentrations of oxygen are a specific antidote. Other drugs such as *chlorpromazine and other phenothiazines* may cause apparent unconsciousness and hypothermia is characteristic. The arrhythmias associated with *tricyclic antidepressants* make careful monitoring essential (*see* 'Poisoning,' p. 193).

Status epilepticus

If a patient does not recover consciousness following an epileptiform seizure a further fit is anticipated and an intravenous cannula inserted for the administration of diazepam.

Gastrointestinal haemorrhage

Patients will present with dizziness or syncope followed by a malaena stool, or perhaps with vomiting of fresh blood, or with fresh blood passed per rectum.

Haematemesis and malaena

Fresh blood in the vomit and black stools both suggest upper gastrointestinal bleeding. The significance of the bleeding is not always easy to determine from the patient's account and management is chiefly based on a sound clinical assessment.

The presence of shock signifies decompensation and a blood sample is sent for grouping and cross-matching of, say, 6 units of blood, and haematocrit estimation. Venous cannulation with a wide bore needle is secured and fluid replacement commenced before the patient is systematically examined.

If, however, the patient appears well and cannot produce evidence of blood at either end of the gastrointestinal tract, he may nevertheless have bled from, for example, a Mallory-Weiss tear induced by vomiting and may bleed again severely. He should therefore be admitted for endoscopy.

Unless the bleeding is so unremitting as to demand urgent surgery, endoscopic diagnosis is the next step and the specialist team is informed.

Rectal bleeding

This symptom produces considerable alarm in the patient but is most commonly due to simple haemorrhoids and the patient can be reassured and instructed to keep his stool soft. Only exceptionally will a mass be palpable to the examining finger. Profuse bleeding is usually associated with pre-existing bowel disorders such as ulcerative colitis or localized lesions such as Meckel's or colonic diverticulae, or a mucosal vascular malformation.

Proctoscopy allows bleeding haemorrhoids to be located and advice should then be sought about possible injection treatment either immediately or in an out-patient clinic. Other causes will require in-patient investigation under the appropriate team.

Poisoning and drug-induced emergencies

Poisoning

The majority of instances of poisoning seen will be *self-inflicted* injuries. The patient is typically a young female adult, but young teenagers, of both sexes, and those in early middle-age are also represented. Children, particulary the toddler, will be the subject of *accidental* poisoning, usually by household products, or family medicines, or botanical specimens.

Management falls into five stages.

Resuscitation

The patient who has made a serious attempt on his or her life with barbiturates, tricyclic antidepressants, dextropropoxyphene, salicylates, paracetamol or narcotics is likely to need urgent airway protection and ventilatory support.

If the patient is unconscious:

1. Secure the airway.
2. Define the level of consciousness.
3. Measure the adequacy of ventilation.
4. Record the pulse, blood pressure, and temperature, if necessary with a low-reading thermometer.

If the patient is conscious he may still be seriously poisoned by, for example, aspirin or paracetamol or tricyclic drugs and he may deteriorate rapidly. He therefore requires urgent treatment with specific measures in order to prevent life-threatening organ damage.

Resuscitative measures may be required in these commonly encountered cases:

1. The barbiturate overdose. The patient's conscious level is profoundly depressed, and it may appear that breathing has virtually ceased. If ventilation is measured by a Wright spirometer and is found to be less than 4 l/min, assisted respiration is likely to be needed and blood gas analysis is performed. Oxygen is administered and intravenous fluids are started. A blood level of the drug is obtained, and if the stomach is to be washed out an endotracheal tube is first inserted.
2. Tricyclic antidepressant drug overdosage may produce alarming and early arrhythmias, and cardiac monitoring is begun immediately.
3. The patient who has taken dextropropoxyphene or other opiates may suffer rapid respiratory arrest.
4. Both paracetamol and salicylate in massive overdosage, if recognition is delayed, will cause life-threatening acidosis and require metabolic correction as a primary measure, as well as cardiorespiratory support.
5. 'Glue-sniffing' and allied adventures are now an occasional cause of seriously ill patients in whom intensive supportive measures may be required.

Identification

Most cases of poisoning seen in Accident and Emergency departments do not require resuscitation and the causal drug or substance is usually known. Where the agent is unknown, the circumstances and the clinical picture can be expected to yield the required information in the majority of cases.

It is possible to identify certain drugs in plasma such as alcohol, iron, salicylates and paracetamol, and these tests should always be carried out if there is any possibility of them being responsible, both to identify the poison and also to quantify the level, as this will affect management. Barbiturate and tricyclic drug levels can also be determined in the blood but this does not affect management as such patients are managed on the basis of their clinical state alone. As these tests take up a considerable amount of time, the laboratory are naturally reluctant to perform them unnecessarily.

Stomach washings and urine samples can be kept for analysis in case of legal consequences.

Few drugs are amenable in fact to specific antagonists and so with the above exceptions no attempt is usually made to investigate further and the patient is treated on general principles dictated by the clinical features.

Elimination

There are four principle methods available:

1. *Gastric lavage and emesis.* Almost all drugs involved will have been absorbed after 6 hours from the time of ingestion, probably well before that time. Therefore if the interval is longer there is no point in subjecting the patient to the procedure. If, however, there is some doubt about the time, you should play safe and empty the stomach. In particular, salicylates, and also tricyclic and phenothiazine drugs are recoverable from gastric washing many hours after ingestion and in these instances lavage, however delayed, should always be insisted on.

   The stomach should *not* be washed out, however, after ingestion of corrosive material such as paraquat, or volatile substances such as petrol, due to the risk of aspiration pneumonitis.

   If the patient has no reliable cough reflex then an anaesthetist must be requested to insert an endotracheal tube and to stand by while the procedure is carried out.

An alternative in children is to administer Syrup of Ipecacuanha (15 ml in 200 ml water) which usually provides satisfactory emesis. Activated charcoal is promoted as a means of reducing absorption of the drug but it is still used as an adjunct to, rather than a replacement for, lavage or induced vomiting.

2. *Forced diuresis.* This is used when the drug is excreted mainly unchanged and is minimally protein bound. It is, in fact, only routinely used in salicylate poisoning, if the blood level exceeds 50 mg/ml, but it can also be used to help eliminate long-acting barbiturates and amphetamines.

3. *Dialysis.* Haemodialysis has a place in the treatment of patients with paraquat poisoning and in some patients severely poisoned with salicylates and long-acting barbiturates.

4. *Haemoperfusion.* Much experimental work is being done on the development of absorbent materials over which blood can be passed, and salicylates and barbiturates can be effectively removed by this means.

Specific measures

There are specific antagonists available for a limited number of poisons and these should be employed in addition to supportive therapy and effective elimination. It is useful to bear in mind the following:

1. Naloxone (Narcan) 0.4 mg intravenously is safe and can be repeated without risk. It is used to counteract *opiates,* including drugs such as codeine and distalgesic, and produces dramatic reversal. However, the dose needs to be repeated at 10 minute intervals, due to its short action, until improvement is maintained,

2. N-acetyl cysteine (Parvolex) is given by intravenous injection in cases of *paracetamol* poisoning, if within 15 hours of ingestion. A dose of 150 mg/kg body weight is given over 15 minutes followed by an infusion at a rate dependent upon blood level monitoring.

3. In life-threatening *alcohol* intoxication 500 ml of 40% fructose given intravenously will help and this can be followed by dextrose solution to correct hypoglycaemia.

4. Physostigmine 2 mg is given when atropine-like manifestations in *antidepressant* poisoning are severe. Fits will require diazepam, and arrhythmias may require lignocaine or other anti-dysrhythmic drugs.

5. Desferrioxamine 5 g placed in the stomach before and after washout is vital in the dangerous poisoning by *iron* tablets commonly seen in children. It can be given parenterally also, if the blood level exceeds 90 mmol/l.
6. Atropine is indicated in *organo-phosphorus insecticide* poisoning.
7. Intravenous cobalt tetracemate 40 mg is used in the treatment of *cyanide* poisoning.
8. Glucagon is given intravenously (5 mg or 3 mg/hour by infusion) when β-*blocking drugs* are the cause. Alternative drugs are isoprenaline or adrenaline.

In all instances there is exact information and advice available from one of the Poison Information Centres by telephone (*see* Appendix I).

Further management

The generally accepted rule is that all patients with self-inflicted poisoning should be admitted for psychiatric assessment even if their medical state does not occasion concern, or require treatment. There will be obvious exceptions to this, but care must be taken not to ignore the truly depressed patient, or to miss serious psychiatric disturbance because of concentration upon the medical aspect. Patients who show drug dependence require separate referral to a specialist treatment centre.

Drug-induced emergencies

Drug reactions

These are common. Many seen in Accident and Emergency departments are manifested by skin rashes, gastrointestinal upset and other minor symptoms, but dangerous anaphylaxis can also occur.

Dystonic drug reactions with muscular spasms causing distressing contortions particularly of the face occur alarmingly frequently with products such as metaclopramide (Maxalon) and phenothiazine derivatives. These are easily reversed by an anticholinergic drug such as benztropine 4 mg by mouth, or procyclidine 10 mg by intravenous injection. The recovery is dramatic.

Anaphylaxis with penicillin, antisera or radio-opaque contrast material is well recognized. The patient may collapse with profound hypotension, or bronchospasm, or may develop airway embarrassment due to pharangeal swelling. The onset may be less dramatic, with urticarial lesions. Management is as follows:

1. Secure the airway. Endotracheal intubation or even cricothyroidotomy (*see* Chapter 25) may be promptly required.
2. Give high concentrations of oxygen.
3. Treat bronchospasm with salbutamol.
4. Give 100 mg hydrocortisone intravenously, and 0.5 ml 1:1000 adrenaline intramuscularly.

Drug reactions

Care should be taken when prescribing drugs, particularly when any existing medication is unknown. Specific problems which commonly occur are with patients who are on warfarin, steroids, or those addicted to alcohol, and a drug interaction chart should be on display in the department.

Hypothermia

Although most commonly encountered amongst the elderly in cold weather, hypothermia is also associated with some drug overdosage, alcohol intoxication, unconsciousness for any other reason, and immersion in water.

The patient may appear to be dead. The temperature measured rectally by a low-reading thermometer may be well below 30°C. However the patient should not automatically be declared dead without senior advice, and intially careful resuscitation should be attempted.

1. Administer oxygen via a secure airway, but do not pass an endotracheal tube unless necessary as the procedure may precipitate arrhythmia.
2. Give intravenous fluids at normal body temperature through a blood warmer. Central venous pressure monitoring is wise, particularly in the elderly.
3. Cover the patient with a 'space' blanket in a warm room. Do not warm actively by immersion in warm water or by peritoneal lavage with warmed fluids unless senior advice is first sought.
4. An ECG, electrolyte and urea estimations, and if necessary arterial blood gas analysis should be performed. The vital signs are monitored regularly. Acidosis may need correction.
5. The patient will need to be handled gently, and unnecessary movement should be avoided.

Drowning

The problems associated with immersion may not simply be due to the inhalation of salt or fresh water. There may well have been an injury, either before or after the fall, and there may be alcohol or other drug-taking to complicate the matter. There may well be resulting hypothermia, and cardiac arrest or dysrhythmias may occur due to sudden exposure to cold water.

Management in the case of cardiac or respiratory arrest is as for other causes. No attempt is made to remove fluid from the bronchial tree unless accessible to a suction catheter. If fluid has been inhaled pulmonary oedema, particularly with salt water, may develop rapidly and a base-line chest X-ray, blood gas estimation, and ECG are required immediately. The possibility of delayed development of pulmonary complications means that if there is any likelihood that water has been inhaled the patient should be admitted for serial observations.

Electrocution

Patients will often present with distress after an electric shock in a domestic or industrial situation when no apparent damage has been caused. If there is undue apprehension, or any residual muscle spasm, or any ECG abnormalities, such a patient should be admitted for a limited period of observation.

If the patient is unconscious he may be in ventricular fibrillation or cardiac standstill. As these patients are normally healthy and often young, resuscitation is pursued optimistically for prolonged periods despite lack of response.

Chapter 24

The accident officer and the law

The junior doctor starting to work in an Accident and Emergency Department is always worried about the legal problems. Apart from his own position and the difficulties in which he may find himself as a result of his own errors of omission or commission, the complexities of the law in relation to his patients are always a source of anxiety. He feels vulnerable in respect of complaints which may be made, sometimes without good grounds, and unless help from more experienced doctors is readily available, he tends to practise defensive medicine by X-raying patients unnecessarily or bringing them back for review at unnecessarily short intervals.

Negligence

The possibility of being sued for negligence is very much in the forefront of the junior's concern, yet it is a situation which applies to all doctors during their clinical work and, even in the casualty situation, should not be allowed to influence the treatment of a patient. Negligence can be defined as: 'a failure to use reasonable skill and care, when treating a patient, which results in damage to that patient'. Once a doctor starts to treat a patient, he undertakes to use reasonable skill and care. The law recognizes that no doctor can have a high degree of skill in every specialty, and therefore the standard of care depends on the experience and position held by the doctor. From this it follows that the junior doctor in an Emergency Department will not be expected to possess the knowledge and experience of the consultant in charge of the department. As a hypothetical example, a junior doctor missing a dislocated lunate bone would not be held to exhibit the degree of negligence that the consultant would display if he missed the same injury.

The defence against negligence is not very simple, but basically requires that the doctor should take a good history, make an adequate examination and **record** his findings and treatment in sufficient detail to enable the situation to be reconstructed at a later date. (These notes should also be decipherable without calling in a handwriting expert.)

Reference has previously been made in earlier chapters to the importance of adequate documentation. The annual reports of the defence societies highlight the problems that are raised by a failure in documentation and, if a doctor is sued for negligence, a defence is only possible if the notes, made at the time or very shortly thereafter, can be produced to support the treatment or advice given to the patient. When the mechanics of the injury, given in the history, and the examination do not suggest that a fracture is present, provided the reasons for not X-raying the patient are clearly set out, a good defence against negligence is possible. In contrast, a single-line comment on the record, without an adequate (and relevant) history or examination, made in an illegible and unsigned scrawl, cannot be regarded as an adequate assessment of the patient and would be of little help in defending an allegation of negligence.

Many complaints and legal interventions are made a considerable time after the patient attended hospital. In a department which sees many thousands of patients every year, the written record is the only adequate means of protecting both the doctor and the patient. Memory under these circumstances is totally unreliable.

It is also good practice to record any untoward or unusual incident that happens to a patient. Legal action against doctors is comparatively rare, but complaints can be a source of considerable worry and it is always best to record full details of incidents while they are fresh in one's memory.

The defence societies, whose membership is compulsory for all National Health Service medical and dental staff, should always be contacted either by telephone or in writing immediately a doctor becomes aware that he is likely to be involved in a complaint or legal action about his treatment of a patient. They will advise the doctor about ethical matters, the handling of complaints against him, problems arising with the administration and the conditions under which he has to work. When major problems do arise, the junior should seek the help of his consultant who will, if necessary, work closely with the defence society on his junior's behalf.

Complaints

Many complaints, as opposed to legal actions, arise from a failure of the doctor to communicate adequately with the patient. The atmosphere of a busy Accident and Emergency Department is frightening, even to intelligent and responsible persons. Many patients attending Accident and Emergency Departments are of restricted ability and intelligence or are overwhelmed by the circumstances in which they find themselves. The doctor must realize that patients do not react normally under these conditions and he should always deal sympathetically with them and satisfy himself that they appreciate what has happened, what treatment they are to have and what arrangements have been made for follow-up. These details should always be entered into the notes in case enquiries are made in the future.

Violence

The aggressive patient does raise difficulties. The doctor should restrain his natural tendencies to reply in kind. Aggression begets aggression and if a sympathetic approach, possibly helped by a member of the nursing staff, is adopted, most patients will quieten down and allow themselves to be treated in the normal way. However, if a patient becomes violent, abusive or aggressive, causes a hazard to other patients or the staff and refuses to leave the department, the police should be asked to remove the offender.

Care must be taken to establish, as far as possible, that such a patient is not suffering from a medical or surgical condition, e.g. hypoglycaemia or a head injury which requires treatment; this group of patients are not responsible for their actions and should be treated appropriately. The uncontrollable drunk, however, may create a dangerous situation for other patients and, if he is not amenable to reason, it is preferable that he should be removed by the police if he will not remove himself. Treatment can always be given when he has sobered up.

Violent patients except, for example, hypoglycaemic cases, should never be given any drugs to control their violence. To do so without their permission will constitute an assault. Of more significance, however, is the danger of giving a patient a powerful drug without any knowledge of any other drugs they may have consumed. The doctor should always be aware that physical restraint of a patient is illegal and whenever this is necessary he should be fully prepared to justify this action.

Refusal of treatment

If a patient refuses to accept treatment or admission to hospital, he must be allowed to discharge himself, preferably after signing an appropriate form accepting the responsibility for his action. If he will not sign such a form, this should be indicated on the case sheet, which must be counter-signed by a witness, who may be either another doctor or a senior nurse. When a person under 16 refuses to accept treatment, the parents should be contacted and asked to attend the department.

When parents refuse to allow essential treatment, e.g. blood transfusion or an operation, to be carried out on a child, possibly for religious reasons, the consultant in charge should be contacted as it may be necessary to take the child into the care of the local authority. In a true emergency situation, resulting from haemorrhage, immediate blood replacement must take precedence over attempts to institute care proceedings before transfusion.

Consent for operation

A standard form is in use in most hospitals for this purpose. It is important that the reason for any surgical procedure should be explained to the patient by the doctor. The doctor advises the patient and it is the patient's privilege to accept or reject this advice. Whenever possible, some idea of the future course of the condition should be given to the patient before the procedure is carried out. The patient knows what to expect and, if a perfect result is unlikely, the patient will accept this more easily if he is aware of the position from the beginning.

Persons over the age of 16 can sign their own consent form but, whenever possible in young persons, every effort should be made to contact the parents before the operation. If the patient does not wish this to be done, the decision should be accepted if the patient is over 16. Under the age of 16, the person deemed to be in charge of the child, e.g. a school teacher or a scout master if the child is away at camp, can sign the consent for operation if it is not practical to contact the parents in time.

In cases of extreme urgency, e.g. an extradural haemorrhage, the doctor must be prepared to carry out the necessary treatment even without permission being obtained. This situation is fortunately not common, but it can occur, particularly after road traffic accidents and, if delay in obtaining parental consent would jeopardize the well-being of the patient, the doctor would be failing in his duty to the patient by accepting such a delay in carrying out the treatment. Equally, there is no urgency when treating closed fractures without circulatory or neurological complications and such patients can be given holding treatment, e.g. splints and sedation until proper consent is obtained.

Confidentiality

The medical profession is privileged by being given information from patients that they would not make available to any other person. In return, patients are entitled to have this confidential information about themselves held under secure conditions and not made available to third persons without their consent. The rule of secrecy may have to be broken when statutory requirements, such as the notification of infectious diseases or the certification of death, have to be completed.

With the patient's permission, information may be disclosed to any third party, such as an employer. When a solicitor acting on behalf of the patient requests information, permission is implied, but a report should never be given to a solicitor or insurance company who does not act for the patient without written permission being obtained. In a Court of Law confidential information about the patient may have to be given if the judge directs that the doctor disclose such information. As a result of the McIver decision made in May 1978 in the House of Lords and the provisions of the Supreme Court Act 1981, if a plaintiff or his solicitor supplies appropriate reasons to a court, they can obtain an order for the disclosure of the hospital records directly to the solicitor. This decision is of importance to the doctor working in an Emergency Department. It emphasizes the necessity to keep good, accurate, legible records and indirectly highlights the need to avoid writing any derogatory comments on the notes which might reflect adversely on his colleagues or on the patient.

If any comments are considered necessary, they should always take the form of factual observations. The use of two- or three-word opinions should be avoided because the doctor would be unlikely to remember the grounds on which he based his opinion by the time the case reached court, and there is also a possibility that a conclusion—as opposed to an observation—might turn out to be wrong. A situation of this nature would reflect little credit on the doctor and could well prejudice the outcome of any proceedings in which he had been asked by the plaintiff or the defendant to give medical evidence.

The rule of confidentiality also extends to specimens taken from the patient. For example, vomit must not be given to the police for forensic examination without the patient's consent, nor must blood samples be taken for the police. In general, the safest approach to the problem of confidentiality is not to give out any information about the patient without his or her permission. This generalization holds good for the majority of circumstances and, when in doubt, the doctor should ask his consultant.

There are two areas where problems can arise, usually unexpectedly, and rapid decisions may have to be made:

1. The Press ring up to enquire about patients who have been injured after accidents. If the injuries are the result of a road traffic accident, it is wisest to refer the enquirer to the police to obtain the information. If the injuries have followed industrial or other accidents, the hospital administration, during the daytime, should be asked to deal with the enquiry. At nights, or when the administration is not available, provided the relatives have been notified a generalized statement as to the patient's condition and injuries can be given. Specific details of the injuries should be avoided and the doctor should not be persuaded by a highly skilled enquirer to enlarge upon the minimal details.

   If several victims have been admitted following an incident which appears to be newsworthy, there will be considerable press activity and the hospital administration must be prepared to establish an enquiry bureau, irrespective of the day or time.

2. Police enquiries after road traffic accidents are necessary, *inter alia,* for statistical purposes and there is no harm in giving appropriate details. If the patient's condition is serious, apart from being prepared to assist in notifying relatives, it may be necessary for further enquiries to be made into the cause of the accident.

When a patient has been seriously assaulted, it may be necessary, provided the time can be spared from the clinical situation, to discuss the injuries with the senior officer in charge of the case. Rapid action by the police may result in the speedy arrest of the assailant and, when the patient's injuries are serious or liable to result in death or serious incapacity, the community has a right to expect that all possible steps will be taken to apprehend a suspect. If the patient's condition permits, it may be necessary to allow the police to have a short interview with the patient; they are always co-operative in these cases and will limit their interview to the length of time allowed by the doctor.

If the injured patient is the alleged assailant or is likely to be charged with a serious offence, the police will insist on one of their officers remaining with the patient at all times. This requirement must be accepted by the staff; it can, if the patient is violent, be of considerable assistance to them in controlling the situation with minimal risk to other patients, staff and equipment.

Drug addicts

Patients suffering from an overdose of any drug of addiction are ill and should be treated appropriately, if necessary by admission.

The registered drug addict who obtains his opiate drugs from a special clinic and comes to the department with withdrawal symptoms, or claiming he has lost or broken his ampoule of morphia or heroin, should be handled sympathetically but carefully. There is a ready market for these drugs and, whenever possible, the Drug Addiction Clinic should be contacted. In many cases it will be found that the alleged story does not stand up and the advice of the clinic should be acted upon.

If the patient is suffering from acute withdrawal symptoms, an injection of methadone may be given and the patient advised to report back to the next available clinic. If such patients keep coming back with differing stories as to how they lost their drugs, or if the number of addicts begins to show a progressive increase, the doctor must consider whether or not he is handling the situation in the correct manner and advice should be obtained from his consultant.

When a young person under 16 is brought into hospital under the influence of drugs, the necessary treatment should be given. The relatives or guardian should be interviewed. If the drugs were obtained from home, appropriate advice should be given about the care of the drugs and the assistance of the general practitioner and, possibly, a psychiatrist sought for the further management of the problem. If the drugs were obtained illegally, the parents should be advised to discuss the matter with the police drug squad, who are very anxious to trace drug pushers and are quite prepared to discuss the problem with the parents without taking any action against the patient.

Pethidine addicts are not infrequent. They may present as cases of renal colic and, on examination, the abdomen often shows external evidence of previous surgery. Usually they arrive late at night and frequently have no local address. It is important not to miss a genuine case and the best approach is to handle them in a fully professional manner. A detailed past history should be obtained, including the names of the last hospitals to which the patient was admitted and the names and addresses of any practitioners the patient has recently consulted. An attempt should be made to contact the hospitals and practitioners by telephone. The information received by such enquiries invariably reveals the genuine case, which contrasts markedly with the lack of information available about the addict. In the latter case the practitioners' names are usually fictitious and there is no record of the patient having been admitted to any of the institutions which he names. When these facts are pointed out to the patient, there is an extremely rapid resolution of the complaints, followed by an equally rapid, voluntary removal of the patient from the department.

Psychiatric problems

Patients with acute psychiatric disorders are often extremely difficult to manage.

The acute hysterical paralysis, while relatively uncommon, is a psychiatric emergency and arrangements should be made for the patient to be seen urgently in a Psychiatric Clinic.

The patient who is determined to commit suicide must never be discharged home. Medical or surgical conditions will require appropriate treatment, but if the Accident and Emergency doctor considers that the patient is seriously considering self-annihilation, he must seek advice from a colleague in the psychiatric department.

When it is considered that the patient has a psychiatric disorder requiring admission to a Mental Hospital the doctor must observe the regulations laid down in the Mental Health Act (1983). Part I of the Act gives the definitions of such terms as: mental disorder, severe impairment, mental impairment and psychopathic disorder. Part II of the Act deals with Compulsory Admission to Hospital. Sections 2, 3 and 4 may be relevant to a situation arising in an Accident and Emergency Department.

Section 2 (formerly *S.25* in the 1959 Act): This section provides for *admission for assessment* for up to 28 days, supported in writing by two registered medical practitioners, on the application of either the nearest relative (defined in Section 26) of the patient, or an approved social worker.

Section 3 (formerly *S.26*) provides for *admission for treatment* on the application of the nearest relative or an approved social worker and with the support of two registered medical practitioners. The detention is (Section 20) for an initial period not exceeding six months (formerly 12 months) renewable after six months for a further six months and, thereafter, at yearly intervals.

Section 4 (*S.29* in the 1959 Act) provides for *emergencies*. In any case of urgent necessity an application for admission may be made either by an approved social worker or by the *nearest* relative of the patient (formerly *any* relative). It must be supported by one medical recommendation given, if practicable, by a practitioner who has previous acquaintance with the patient and it is valid for up to 72 hours. The certifying practitioner must have personally seen the patient within the previous 24 hours.

Legal procedures

The Coroner

Recommendations from a Coroner's Court carry considerable weight and, in the hospital context, can produce speedy action to prevent the recurrence of a situation which would necessitate the holding of an inquest.

The law requires that death occurring under certain circumstances, or from specific diseases, should be reported to the Coroner. To report a death to the Coroner, the details of the death are notified by telephone to the Coroner's Officer, who is usually a Police Officer attached to the Coroner for this purpose. If he should not be available, the death can be reported to the local police station. In certain hospitals, a member of the administrative staff is responsible for such notifications, and it is always wise for the junior doctor to ascertain the local routine for dealing with such matters.

The following deaths should be notified to the Coroner. All cases where death is the result of violence, unnatural causes or is due to natural causes but the doctor cannot certify death because he has not previously treated the patient. Deaths occurring during anaesthesia, as a result of surgery or attributable to the treatment should also be notified. The Coroner should also be notified of all deaths occurring in mental hospitals, prisons, in persons suffering from prescribed occupational diseases, certain toxic industrial substances and when the person is in receipt of a war pension or pension for an industrial disease.

When the patient dies in the Accident Department, it is the doctor's responsibility to ensure that the Coroner is notified. When the doctor merely confirms death and the body is removed to the mortuary, the responsibility for the notification belongs to the authorities responsible for the mortuary services. However, when death appears to be due to violence inflicted upon the deceased by another person, it is advisable that the police should be notified immediately and instructions given that the body and clothing should not be disturbed in any way, other than to establish that death has occurred.

From time to time the junior doctor will be unsure as to the appropriate action he should take in relation to a death. Staff in A & E Departments should never be required to give a death certificate, although such certificates can be given by the general practitioner who has been looking after the patient. When there is uncertainty, the junior doctor should seek the help of his consultant or ring up the Coroner personally and ask for advice. Usually the Coroner's Officer or clerk will be able to assist and, if not, they will contact the Coroner and ask for his instructions.

If the doctor feels that his conduct is in any way likely to be criticized at an inquest, he should contact his Defence Society immediately. He should also write out a full report on the incident which is causing him concern. Preferably the content of the report should be scrutinized by the Defence Society before submission to either the Coroner or the Hospital Administrator.

Courts

Anyone working in an Accident and Emergency Department comes into frequent contact with the results of personal violence. As a consequence he may be required to make a statement to a Police Officer. This is a formal document setting out the doctor's name, qaulifications and post. It then deals with the facts of the case as known to the doctor and terminates with a conclusion. This may indicate his opinion as to the degree of violence used, the severity of the injury, and an indication that the injuries are compatible with the use of a certain implement or weapon. The statement is then signed by the doctor and a statutory fee will be paid. Junior doctors must avoid being 'carried away' by the supposed drama of the situation and should avoid expressing an opinion on matters which are not commensurate with their professional experience.

The doctor must always keep a copy of his statement because he may subsequently be required to appear in court to be questioned on the statement. Should this happen, he will be notified by the police of the time and date of the hearing. On arrival at court he should report to the usher, if he is not recognized by the Constable involved, who will advise him where he can wait until his case is due to be heard. When he is required to give evidence, he enters the witness box and takes the oath to speak the truth in a manner appropriate to his religious belief.

He will then be taken through his statement by the prosecutor, who may be either a Police Officer or a solicitor. He will then be asked questions by the defence solicitor. It is important that his evidence is given clearly, and it should be addressed to the

Magistrates. The doctor should never hesitate, if skilled question-ing draws a false conclusion, to indicate that, in his view, the conclusion is erroneous. It is equally important to confine his comments to matters about which he is confident. Solicitors are skilled in the art of cross-examination and the inexperienced doctor can find himself in a situation where he is admitting that what he has just said in evidence is not really as accurate as he had imagined before he made his comments.

If the crime is of greater magnitude than can be dealt with by Magistrates, it will be heard in the Crown Court. This is a court presided over by a judge with a jury, where the examination and cross-examination is carried out by barristers. The doctor's statement will be taken on a special form; it may be typed out on the form and he will have to sign each page. The evidence is initially heard by Magistrates at committal proceedings, where the decision is made that the nature of the crime demands that the accused be sent to the Crown Court for trial. The doctor is not usually required to attend these proceedings.

He will later be given a subpoena, that is a legal document requiring him to attend the court and give evidence in the case of Regina v. the accused. This document must not be ignored and the courts are always sympathetic if there are times when a doctor cannot attend, provided that the problem has been discussed in good time. The police are the appropriate persons to contact if there are any difficulties, such as examinations, likely to arise at about the time of the hearing.

The procedure in court follows a similar, though a slightly more formal, course to that in the Magistrates' Court. The evidence should be given clearly and directed towards the judge and jury. Barristers are even more skilled than solicitors in putting words in the mouths of inexperienced doctors and the only sound advice is to answer the questions simply and never volunteer any information. If you do not know or are doubtful about the answer to a question, say so.

Despite the rather worrying surroundings, the whole procedure is conducted quietly and with great politeness. The judge is, in some ways, in a position of a referee and, if the questioning appears to be getting unreasonable, or if the conclusions drawn by the barristers are inaccurate, the fact should be made known to the judge.

Judges are addressed as 'My Lord' or 'Your Honour'. The former applies to a High Court Judge who is on circuit, i.e. taking the serious cases in the courts around the circuit. The latter applies to a less senior judge, who spends his time entirely in a restricted number of courts, hearing all but the most serious cases. Occasionally a recorder, who is a barrister 'acting up' as a judge may take the case. The precise mode of address can be ascertained by listening to the barristers when they address the judge. Magistrates are addressed as 'Sir' or 'Madam'.

Even in Crown Court proceedings, the junior doctor will be acting as a witness to fact. An expert witness is usually a senior member of the profession with special skills in a certain field who has been asked to study and comment about the medical evidence. Such a witness may be used by both the prosecution and defence, and the junior should feel relieved that the barristers reserve their main attacks for these persons.

Drinking and driving

When the driver of a motor vehicle is brought to hospital for examination and treatment after an accident, the Police Officer in charge of the case may request permission to 'breathalyse' the patient. Once the patient has entered the Accident and Emergency department the Police Officer is not allowed to perform this investigation without the permission of the doctor who is treating the patient. The doctor will usually give permission and should record the fact on the record card. Current legislation states that the patient may be charged with an offence if the level of alcohol exceeds $35 \mu g/100 ml$ of breath when a Lion Intoximeter 3.000 is used. Often leeway is allowed up to $40 \mu g/100 ml$ before prosecution automatically follows. For breath levels up to $50 \mu g/100 ml$ the patient can request that a blood sample be taken in the hope that this will show that the blood level is below $80 mg$ of alcohol per $100 ml$ of blood. Or, if the patient requests it, a sample of urine can be analysed, the critical level being $107 mg$ of alcohol in $100 ml$ of urine.

As with the breath sample, blood or urine samples can only be taken in hospital with the doctor's permission, and with the patient's permission. The Accident and Emergency doctor, having given permission, is then in no way involved in the taking or analysing of the samples. The Police Officer or the Police Surgeon will take the samples and they must not use any of the hospital's equipment in the process nor will the hospital be involved in the analysis.

The doctor must give permission if the patient's condition would not be adversely affected by the procedure. It should be refused if the patient is unconscious or suffering from injuries which would prevent the test being carried out. These include facial or chest injuries which would prevent the breathalyser bag being blown up during expiration. Severe shock, haemorrhage or major injuries would also be contraindications. The presence of other injuries does not preclude the test.

If permission for the test is refused by the doctor, the matter is closed. If it is considered that the patient is fit to undergo the test, the doctor should explain to the patient: 'This Officer has asked me if he can carry out a breathalyser test on you. In my opininon you are fit to undergo the test and I have given him my permission to approach you for this purpose. He will explain the law to you, as I have no further involvement in the matter'.

Despite the apparent simplicity of the procedure, the doctor may still find himself in court giving evidence for the defence or prosecution, and certain precautions are advisable to avoid this happening.

When the patient refuses the provision of a blood sample, if the breathalyser is positive he may be charged with refusing to provide the specimen and may claim that, because of his injuries, he was not aware of what he was doing. The doctor must, therefore, satisfy himself that the patient is able to understand what was explained to him by the doctor and what was requested by the Police Officer. Clearly, an unconscious or badly confused patient with a head injury will have no understanding, but an inebriated patient may present difficulties from the cognitive aspect. It is advisable that the doctor records his decision about permission or refusal for the test and the reasons for this decision on the case sheet. In this way, if questions of the patient's fitness are raised at a later date by either side, the doctor is in a position to give a reasoned answer to the questions and may avoid the necessity to give evidence in court.

The Accident and Emergency doctor can only have three decisions to make:

1. Is the patient fit or unfit to be interviewed by the Police Officer?
2. Is the patient fit to provide a specimen of breath?
3. Is the patient fit to provide a specimen of blood or urine?

Once these decisions have been made, both the doctor and the hospital have no further part to play and the situation must be resolved between the patient and the Police Officer without outside assistance.

If the Accident and Emergency doctor determines breath, blood or urine alcohol levels to help him in the clinical management of the patient, the results he obtains are not admissable in any legal proceedings and this should be explained to the patient.

Chapter 25

Practical procedures

Intravenous access

Taking a blood sample

This venepuncture is usually performed in the antecubital fossa. If the veins are collapsed, rather than waste time, try the external jugular or the femoral vein. Be sure not to take blood for investigation from an arm in which a 'drip' has been or is running.

Intravenous cannulation

Try to use the forearm veins, or those on the back of the hand, having taken blood first from a proximal vein. If none are accessible the antecubital fossa will have to be used for this also. Do not use the ankle veins if a major abdominal or pelvic injury is suspected.

If unsuccessful, try the external jugular vein. If this is not possible for any reason there are several options left.

Subclavian vein cannulation

This is the preferred site for critically ill patients and the technique should be watched and learnt by every Casualty Officer.

The patient is supine, and the head end of the trolley is tilted down 10–20 degrees. A small sand bag between the shoulders is helpful. The skin is cleaned thoroughly, and drapes are applied to enclose the area. A large bore needle and cannula is inserted 1 cm below and lateral to the mid-point of the (preferably right) clavicle (*Figure 25.1,* A) and is passed medially towards the upper limit of the suprasternal notch passing immediately behind the clavicle (*Figure 25.2*). The needle encounters only slight resistance from the clavi-pectoral fascia and the entry into the subclavian vein is often distinctly felt. The needle is withdrawn and an infusion incorporating a central venous pressure monitor is connected to the cannula.

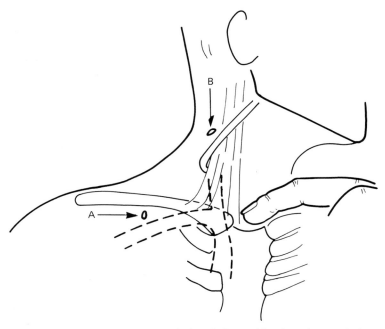

Figure 25.1 A. Subclavian vein cannulation. *B*. Internal jugular vein cannulation

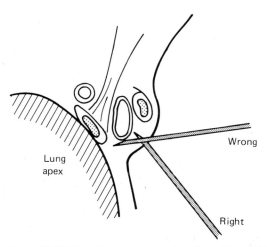

Figure 25.2 Subclavian vein cannulation (keep close behind the clavicle)

Other software is available employing the Seldinger technique: after the needle is introduced, an obturator is threaded into the vein, the needle is withdrawn, and a wide bore cannula is passed over the obturator into the vein; the obturator is finally removed. Alternatively, sets are available that require a cannula to be passed into the vein within the lumen of the needle which is then withdrawn and taped to the skin: the disadvantage here is that it results in a smaller bore cannula having to be used.

The siting of the cannula in the superior vena cava should be confirmed radiographically before fixing securely to the skin.

The Casualty Officer should be familiar with the various items of software used in the department and he should learn to use the materials he finds easiest to handle.

Internal jugular vein cannulation

The patient is positioned as for subclavian venepuncture, and the head is turned away from the side of access (*Figure 25.1, B*). The skin is cleaned and isolated with drapes. The skin is entered at a point two finger-breadths, or 3.5 cm, above the clavicle at the lateral border of the sternomastoid. The needle is advanced towards the suprasternal notch and enters the vein behind the sterno-clavicular joint on the same side.

'Cut-down' cannulation

If the veins are collapsed, or unusable for any reason, and if the Casualty Officer has no experience of subclavian vein or internal jugular vein cannulation, then time must not be wasted. This is particularly relevant with infants and small children. Proceed immediately to approach anatomically predictable and accessible veins by incision and cannulation under direct vision. A pack should be available to hand which contains a small (No. 15 blade) scalpel, fine sharp dissecting scissors, fine dissecting forceps and several fine artery forceps. Swabs and a perforated drape will also be required.

Following rapid skin preparation, and infiltration of local anaesthetic if necessary, an incision is made over the median cubital vein, or the cephalic vein in the antecubital fossa, or the long saphenous vein 2 cm anterior to the medial malleolus, or the same vein in the groin 3 cm below and lateral to the pubic tubercle.

After exposure of the vein it can be entered in the usual way with a large bore needle and cannula which is either introduced through the skin distal to the wound (*Figure 25.3*) or through the vein in the wound directly. A long cannula can be introduced directly if a small cut is made in the vein wall with the point of the scissors.

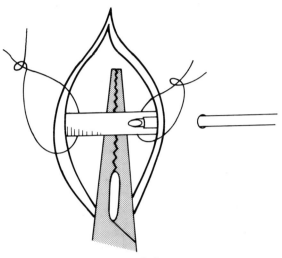

Figure 25.3 'Cut-down' cannulation

Scalp vein cannulation

This method is often preferred in neonates and small infants but should not be attempted without first being observed, and if there is any hesitancy, cut-down cannulation should be carried out without delay.

Central venous pressure

The software needed for this should be familiar to the Casualty Officer and a large bore cannula will need to be used. The instructions accompanying the particular equipment used need to be studied and the procedure needs to be rehearsed.

Taking an arterial blood sample

Use the radial artery for preference, or the femoral artery if the former is unavailable. Prepare a heparinized syringe and feel the pulse with the pulp of the non-dominant index finger.

Insert the needle (21G) angulated in the long axis (*Figure 25.4*) to pass into the artery beneath the examining finger. The pulse will be felt at the needle point before entry.

As the blood is withdrawn check that it looks arterial, and after withdrawal of the needle maintain digital pressure over the site for three minutes by the clock.

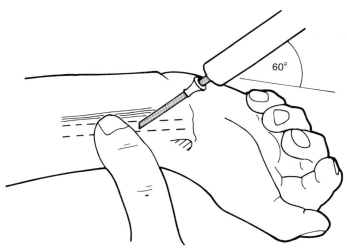

Figure 25.4 Taking an arterial blood sample

Intercostal drain insertion

There are two sites in common use.

1. The second intercostal space is entered in the mid-clavicular line. This is used primarily for pneumothorax, and in particular as an urgent measure in tension pneumothorax.

   The patient is propped up as far as is comfortable and the skin is cleaned and local anaesthetic infiltrated. The area is screened with drapes and a small incision made through the full thickness of the chest wall. A medium sized (24 Fr) trocar and cannula are introduced and the cannula clamped as the trocar is withdrawn. The cannula is then connected to an underwater seal, or a flutter valve, and unclamped. Air should bubble out of the tube with each expiration, and the quantity of any fluid that drains out should be measured.

In the exceptional emergency of a tension pneumothorax an intravenous needle and cannula can be inserted immediately at the same site and the air under tension allowed to equalize with the atmosphere as a temporary measure.

2. The second site is at the 5th or 6th intercostal space in the mid-axillary line. This is the preferred site for a number of reasons. It does not leave a scar in a conspicuous place, and thus a large bore tube (28–32 Fr) can be used. It is more appropriate for drainage of both fluid and air in a recumbent patient. It is not so painful to put in, and patients find it more comfortable afterwards.

Peritoneal lavage

This is the best way at present to determine the presence of intra-abdominal bleeding. However, this investigation should not be embarked on without the agreement of the admitting surgical team.

The steps are as follows:

1. Catheterize the bladder.
2. Infiltrate the abdominal skin down to peritoneum two fingers breadth below the umbilicus with local anaesthetic.
3. Make a small incision.
4. Introduce a dialysis trocar and cannula into the peritoneal cavity aiming towards the pelvis, withdraw the trocar, and attach an infusion set to the cannula from a 1 litre bag of saline.
5. Allow the saline to run in unchecked. It should run easily. Look for any evidence of extraperitoneal extravasation. When the bag is empty, move the patient gently from side to side. After one minute, allow the fluid to run out again by lowering the bag to floor level.

A significant amount of blood staining of the effluent indicates the need for exploration. Contraindications to this procedure are pregnancy or a previous laparotomy.

Pericardial aspiration

The patient is propped up if possible. The most useful site of puncture is at the xiphisternum, and the area is thoroughly cleaned and draped. Local anaesthetic is introduced to all layers of the abdominal wall, and then a long intravenous needle and cannula are introduced in the left costo-xiphoid angle and angled upwards at 45° to the vertical to traverse the abdominal musculature and to enter the pericardium above the diaphragm (*Figure 25.5 (a)* and (*b*)). There is usually a distinctive sensation when the pericardium is punctured and positive aspiration will confirm correct positioning. Following removal of the needle, aspiration is continued through the cannula and clinical improvement should be immediately obvious.

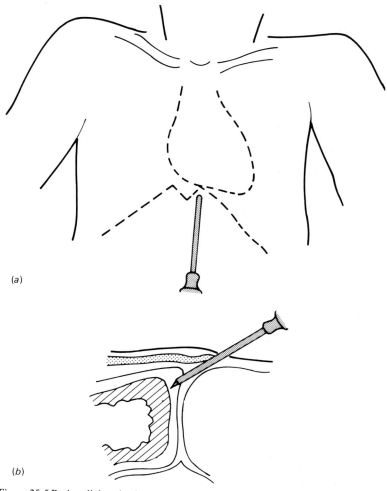

(a)

(b)

Figure 25.5 Pericardial aspiration

Tracheotomy

The requirement for urgent direct access to the trachea is rare in Accident and Emergency work in this country. Normally there will be time to arrange for formal tracheostomy under ideal conditions by specialist staff. Emergency tracheotomy as described in text books using a knife and a variety of devices to open an airway into the trachea is far too hazardous to undertake, and should not be attempted now that a safe and easy method is available.

Cricothyroid stab

1. Position the patient with a pillow under the shoulders to extend the neck.
2. Grasp the thyroid cartilage with the non-dominant hand between finger and thumb (*Figure 25.6*).
3. Insert a large intravenous needle and cannula (Size 12 or larger) through the cricothyroid membrane vertically and withdraw the needle. This should provide sufficient airflow, but if not, another cannula can be inserted beside it. Attach an adaptor and connect to a ventilator if necessary.
4. Ask for urgent specialist help to perform formal tracheostomy.

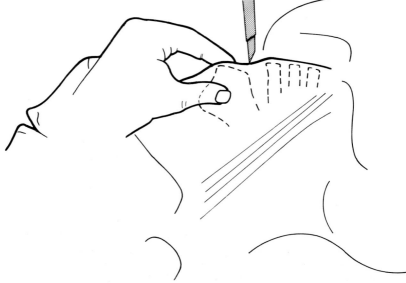

Figure 25.6 Cricothyroid stab

The bleeding tooth socket

A common dental emergency is the patient who is bleeding from the socket of a tooth removed earlier that same day. The bleeding occurs, not from the socket, but from the edge of the alveolar mucosa around the rim of the socket. If a dentist is not available, follow this procedure:

1. Get the patient to bite on a pad soaked in adrenaline solution which has been laid in the socket. A full 5 minutes pressure should be encouraged.

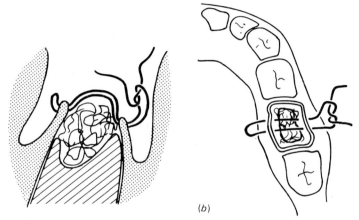

(a)   (b)

Figure 25.7 The bleeding tooth socket may be sutured together by a mattress stitch over a dental roll which has plugged the socket

2. If this is unsuccessful, the gum margins can be sutured together by a mattress stitch over a dental roll which has plugged the socket (*Figure 25.7*). This controls the bleeding by pressing the mucosa against the bony socket. This is retained until the patient sees his dentist the following day (*Figures 25.8(a)* and (*b*)).

Control of epistaxis

The usual site of bleeding is Kiesselbach's plexus of vessels in Little's area, the area of the septum that you see on lifting the alar. If the bleeding has stopped and the point of origin obvious, it can be cauterized immediately by touching the bleeding point with the tip of a silver nitrate stick.

If the bleeding continues, control is achieved by simple thumb and forefinger pressure for 5 minutes. If bleeding recurs persistently, despite prolonged periods of pressure, packing is carried out. The nasal cavity is sprayed with 4% cocaine or 10% xylocaine solution, or a cotton bud soaked in 10% cocaine and 1:1000 adrenaline is placed in the nose. There are then a number of options:

1. Anterior nasal packing can be performed with 0.5 in ribbon gauze soaked in BIPP ointment (*Figure 25.8(a)*). Pick up the gauze with sinus forceps 5 cm from the end and insert it, doubled, horizontally along the floor of the nose to the posterior limit of the cavity. Pick up the next length 5 cm from the external nares, and thus build up layers from the floor up to the roof, finally leaving an obvious loose end free at the nostril (*Figure 25.8(b)*). This can remain in place for up to 48 hours before removal in an ENT clinic.
2. Balloon catheters are now available, although expensive, and are simple to insert and inflate.
3. Nasal tampons are also useful as a rapid and comfortable way of exerting presure locally and are less expensive than balloons.

The bleeding may occur from the posterior portion of the nasal cavity, most commonly in the older person, and associated with hypertension. Even if bleeding has ceased by the time the patient is seen, a haemoglobin estimation and a cardiovascular examination is wise.

If bleeding continues it may be controlled by a balloon catheter, or a long nasal tampon, in the same way as indicated above.

However a posterior nasal pack is sometimes necessary when bleeding is severe and persistent, and the procedure is as follows:

1. Tie ribbon gauze around a dental roll leaving both tails 20 cm long. Repeat with the same dental roll, giving four tails.
2. Thread a soft catheter through the nose, and pull out the tip through the mouth.
3. Tie it to one end of ribbon gauze and pull this back through the nose. Repeat this exercise through the other nostril (*Figure 25.8(c)*).
4. The ends of the ribbon gauze are tied together in front of the columella tight enough to bring the dental roll firmly against the nasal septum. Leave the ribbon gauze in the mouth long, and tape to the corner of the mouth so that the dental roll can be removed easily.

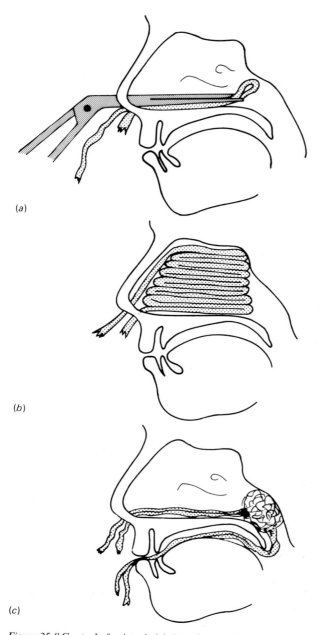

Figure 25.8 Control of epistaxis (*a*) Anterior nasal packing. (*b*) Gauze packed in layers leaving an obvious loose end free at the nostril. (*c*) Posterior nasal pack

5. Pack the nose as described above, pushing the gauze up against the buttress of the dental roll. After 48 hours this can be removed to allow inspection, and if bleeding does not recur the ribbon gauze at the columella is cut and the roll withdrawn through the mouth.

Putting on a plaster cast

The Casualty Officer must be able to apply correctly an appropriate cast following any fracture or joint manipulation he may have carried out. Other staff will generally apply routine casts at other times. (There are now several alternatives to POP on the market but none of these are as useful after manipulation where moulding requires to be done.) The Casualty Officer should practice cast techniques on normal subjects until competent.

1. Plan your cast ahead. Have ready the unwrapped bandages you require and decide whether to use a slab or slabs, or circular bandaging. The slab is easier to use, and for most purposes is adequate as a primary external fixation until the initial swelling diminishes after a few days. It can then be completed, or replaced. Make up the slab(s) to measure before beginning the manipulation.
2. Make sure there is adequate padding to allow for swelling. Compacted wool bandages are universally available and are applied liberally around the fracture site.
3. The purpose is to immobilize the joint above and below the fracture as a rule, although notable exceptions are the routine Colles' fracture and some ankle fractures, where the injury is adjacent to a joint. If two joints are to be encased, deal with one joint at a time, waiting until the first cast is firm enough to support the position gained, before transferring attention to the other joint.
4. After the manipulation make sure the assistant is maintaining the reduction correctly while you apply the cast.
5. Soak the plaster in luke-warm water and squeeze to allow all the air bubbles to escape. Do not squeeze the water out of the cast too enthusiastically in case drying occurs before the cast is complete and smooth and moulded. The colder the water, and the wetter the plaster, the more time you have to make adjustments before it sets. Mould with the flat of the hand and avoid finger indentations.

6. The plaster slab will then be secured with a conforming bandage, better applied thoroughly wet, firmly but not tightly enclosing the limb. Make sure that the ends of this plaster do not restrict joint movement and that there are no sharp edges to cause plaster sores.
7. Always check the position of the fracture by X-ray before the anaesthetic is terminated but after the cast is applied.
8. The cast will take 1–2 days to dry fully, and needs to be protected from undue stress in the meantime. Patients must be given some written instruction about possible complications and proper care for their plasters.

Colles' fracture management

The following procedure is applicable to all adult patients with fractures of the lower end of the radius, with or without fracture of the ulna. It is also applicable to children with a fracture separation of the distal radial epiphysis but it does *not* apply to the completely displaced fracture of the lower end of radius and ulna in a child. This demands a separate procedure, referred to in Chapter 12.

Anaesthesia

When the patient is a child, or is a young adult with a displaced Colles' fracture, it is best to use a general anaesthetic to ensure adequate relaxation.

In other instances, local anaesthetic into the fracture haematoma, or intravenous regional anaesthesia (Bier's Block) are used. Both methods in practised hands give pain-free manipulations.

Intra-fracture analgesia.   The step in continuity of the lateral border of the radius which marks the fracture is easily palpable and is tender. The area is cleaned thoroughly with an iodine skin preparation and the area screened. After scrubbing up, the operator inserts a 23 G needle into the fracture site by entering the skin at an angle 0.5 cm proximal to the fracture at the angle between the extensor pollicis brevis and extensor carpi radialis longus. The fracture is entered by gently working the needle point, angled forwards to conform with the angle of the distal fragment, into the gap between the bone ends (*Figure 25.9*). Entry is confirmed by aspiration of haematoma with the syringe. 10 ml of 1% lignocaine is injected and the fracture rapidly loses its tenderness. The ulnar side of the wrist, if tender, will also need infiltrating similarly, even if no fracture is seen.

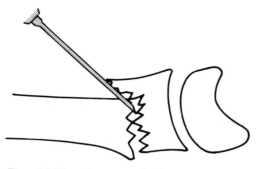

Figure 25.9 Intra-fracture analgesia

As soon as the pain of the fracture on movement disappears, manipulation can be attempted. The attractive feature of this method is its speed, the persisting analgesia, and the predictability of the result if used correctly. The drawback is the lack of muscular relaxation and the patient must be repeatedly encouraged not to resist the procedure and to allow the wrist to relax fully during plaster fixation.

Intravenous regional anaesthesia (IVRA).   Although no complications need be expected, it is wise for full resuscitation measures to be available. The patient is weighed, and the blood pressure measured.

A 19 G butterfly needle or cannula is placed in a vein on the back of the affected hand and secured. The arm is elevated for 3 minutes. A pressure cuff around the upper arm is then elevated to 50 mm Hg above the patient's systolic blood pressure, and the arm placed horizontally. Prilocaine, 30 ml of 0.5% solution (2.5 mg/kg body weight, or 0.6 ml/kg) is slowly injected over 1 minute and 5 minutes are allowed before manipulation is attempted. After the manipulation is complete, the tourniquet must be kept in place for a total of at least 15 minutes to allow fixing of the anaesthetic, before it is deflated. The patient should be allowed to rest under observation for an hour after this procedure.

Manipulation

To reduce the fracture correctly the objective must be clearly understood. Long term problems for these patients usually arise from the shortening of the radius and relative lengthening of the

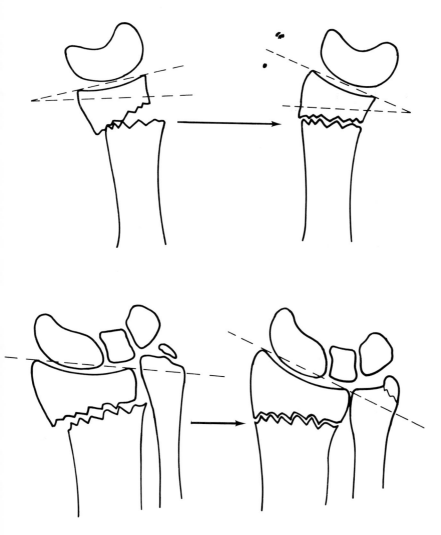

Figure 25.10 Manipulation of Colles' fracture with restoration of normal angles

ulna, producing deformity and disruption of the lower radio-ulnar joint. The object, therefore, must be:

1. To bring the radius out to length.
2. To flex and pronate the distal fragment into its anatomical position. The normal angles of the articular surface of the radius and the relative lengths of the radius and ulna must therefore be restored as precisely as possible (*Figure 25.10*).

The assistant stands by the head of the patient and grasps around the elbow joint, which is flexed to a right angle. The operator grasps the patient's hand with both of his and exerts longitudinal steady traction until he is satisfied that adequate length has been restored. He then moves his dominant hand to place his thenar eminence over the distal fragment of radius, and flexes and pronates the fragment by pushing downwards and ulnarwards. Considerable force may be required, and counter pressure is supplied by the other hand which supports the forearm proximal to the fracture. The patient will then usually allow this position to be maintained simply by allowing the wrist to flex unaided with the elbow supported while the plaster is applied.

The operator applies circular wool bandaging and lays the wet plaster slab on the forearm. It should enclose over half the forearm circumference and should extend to, but not beyond, the metacarpo-phalangeal joints: it should not impede flexion of the elbow joint. Conforming material is used to bandage the slab into place, and while the plaster sets, the reduced position is firmly maintained by the operator.

A post-reduction check radiograph is then taken to confirm a satisfactory position before the anaesthesia is terminated. Finally a high sling is applied to discourage oedema formation in the fingers.

Appendix I

Poison information centres

Cardiff	0222 569200
Dublin	0001 745588
Edinburgh	031 229 2477 Ext. 2233
Leeds	0532 430715
London	01 635 9191
Newcastle	0632 321525

Appendix II

Paediatric data

Total blood volume

Birth	90 ml/kg body weight
1–5 years	80 ml/kg body weight
5 years–adult	70 ml/kg body weight

Weight

At birth	3.5 kg
6 months	7.0 kg
1 year	10.0 kg
2 years	12.0 kg
5 years	18.0 kg
10 years	30.0 kg

Dosage of drugs

Adrenaline Inj. ⎱ 1 in 10 000 ⎰	i.v. 0.1 ml/kg 5 ml maximum
Sodium bicarbonate	2 m.eq/kg SLOWLY
Calcium gluconate	2 ml of 10% SOLUTION
Lignocaine	1 mg/kg (2mg = 0.1 ml of 2% solution)
Phenytoin	3–5 mg/kg SLOWLY
Dexamethasone	0.5–5 mg depending on weight
Diazepam i.v.	0.1 mg/kg SLOWLY, ONCE ONLY
Vallergan	3 mg/kg

Defibrillation

Use 20 Joules for INFANTS
75 Joules for CHILDREN

Endotracheal tubes

6 months	Magill 000 or 00
6 months–1 year	Magill 0
1–2 years	Magill 1
2–6 years	Magill 2 or 3
6–8 years	Magill 4
8–10 years	Magill 5
10–14 years	Magill 6 or 7

Index

233